THE COMPLETE IDIOT'S GUIDE TO

Belly Fat
Weight Loss

by Claire Wheeler, MD, PhD, and Diane A. Welland, MS, RD

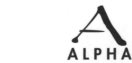

ALPHA

A member of Penguin Group (USA) Inc.

This work is dedicated to my children Eli, Walker, and Jackson with love and gratitude. —Claire

This book is dedicated to my husband Kevin. Thank you for always being there. —Diane

ALPHA BOOKS

Published by the Penguin Group

Penguin Group (USA) Inc., 375 Hudson Street, New York, New York 10014, USA • Penguin Group (Canada), 90 Eglinton Avenue East, Suite 700, Toronto, Ontario M4P 2Y3, Canada (a division of Pearson Penguin Canada Inc.) • Penguin Books Ltd., 80 Strand, London WC2R 0RL, England • Penguin Ireland, 25 St. Stephen's Green, Dublin 2, Ireland (a division of Penguin Books Ltd.) • Penguin Group (Australia), 250 Camberwell Road, Camberwell, Victoria 3124, Australia (a division of Pearson Australia Group Pty. Ltd.) • Penguin Books India Pvt. Ltd., 11 Community Centre, Panchsheel Park, New Delhi—110 017, India • Penguin Group (NZ), 67 Apollo Drive, Rosedale, North Shore, Auckland 1311, New Zealand (a division of Pearson New Zealand Ltd.) • Penguin Books (South Africa) (Pty.) Ltd., 24 Sturdee Avenue, Rosebank, Johannesburg 2196, South Africa • Penguin Books Ltd., Registered Offices: 80 Strand, London WC2R 0RL, England

Copyright © 2012 by Claire Wheeler and Diane A. Welland

International Standard Book Number: 978-1-61564-130-7
Library of Congress Catalog Card Number: 2011908150

14 13 12   8 7 6 5 4 3 2 1

Interpretation of the printing code: The rightmost number of the first series of numbers is the year of the book's printing; the rightmost number of the second series of numbers is the number of the book's printing. For example, a printing code of 12-1 shows that the first printing occurred in 2012.

Printed in the United States of America

Note: This publication contains the opinions and ideas of its authors. It is intended to provide helpful and informative material on the subject matter covered. It is sold with the understanding that the authors and publisher are not engaged in rendering professional services in the book. If the reader requires personal assistance or advice, a competent professional should be consulted.

The authors and publisher specifically disclaim any responsibility for any liability, loss, or risk, personal or otherwise, which is incurred as a consequence, directly or indirectly, of the use and application of any of the contents of this book.

Most Alpha books are available at special quantity discounts for bulk purchases for sales promotions, premiums, fundraising, or educational use. Special books, or book excerpts, can also be created to fit specific needs.

For details, write: Special Markets, Alpha Books, 375 Hudson Street, New York, NY 10014.

Publisher: *Marie Butler-Knight*
Associate Publisher: *Mike Sanders*
Executive Managing Editor: *Billy Fields*
Acquisitions Editor: *Brook Farling*
Development Editor: *Jennifer Bowles*
Senior Production Editor: *Janette Lynn*

Copy Editor: *Tricia Leibig*
Cover Designer: *Kurt Owens*
Book Designers: *William Thomas, Rebecca Batchelor*
Indexer: *Angie Bess Martin*
Layout: *Brian Massey*
Senior Proofreader: *Laura Caddell*

ALWAYS LEARNING   PEARSON

Contents

Introduction

Belly fat. It seems to be everywhere these days—you hear about it on television and read about it in magazines and the papers. But with all this information about belly fat that's out there, it's still hard to know exactly what belly fat is, where it comes from, or how to get rid of it. That's why we've written this book.

Losing belly fat isn't about cutting calories or going to extremes at the gym. Belly fat is a special kind of fat that collects inside your abdomen where you can't see it—but you can tell it's there when your waistline starts expanding. This type of fat buildup has three basic causes:

- Eating too many of the wrong foods

- Not getting enough physical activity each day

- The stress, hassles, and upsets of modern life

Belly fat, more than the fat under your skin that you can pinch, is dangerous to your heart and other organs. It's associated with diabetes, heart disease, high cholesterol, and other problems—so the sooner you get rid of it, the better.

We're going to help you lose your belly fat once and for all. Using the latest scientific and medical information, effective exercise and stress management techniques, and our delicious, satisfying meal plan, you'll be able to trim your middle—but that's not all. You'll also feel better, look better, and have more energy. Your clothes will fit better, you'll feel calmer and less frazzled, and you'll lower your risk of chronic disease.

This isn't a diet—it's a comprehensive plan for your new lifestyle—one that's not about deprivation, but about enjoying, embracing, and appreciating every day. As with any big lifestyle change, it's a good idea to let your doctor know what you're doing—especially if you're over 45, if you have any history of heart disease or other medical issues, or if you haven't exercised for over a year or two.

How This Book Is Organized

This guide has seven parts, each one designed to be simple to understand and easy to use in your everyday life. Our goal is to take you step by step from where you are now—wanting to lose your belly—to where you're headed—leaner, cleaner, and more vital.

Part 1, The Belly Fat Issue, looks at how our modern world can be hazardous to your health. During the past few hundred years, human physiology hasn't changed—but our environment has changed drastically. We eat more, move less, and have more stressful lives than our ancestors did—and we're seeing very high levels of heart disease, diabetes, and obesity as a result. You'll find out exactly what belly fat is, what causes it, and what it does to your health. You'll see some up-to-the-minute research on the connections between stress, your belly, and your health.

Part 2, Your New Food Lifestyle, introduces you to a new way of eating that's enjoyable and satisfying. We'll take a look at the latest research on the ill effects of some types of fat and carbohydrates, and you'll learn which ones to enjoy and what to avoid as you lose your belly. You don't have to exclude carbohydrates from your diet to be lean, you just need to choose wisely. You'll also learn how to include drinks in your lean belly plan.

Part 3, Getting a Handle on Stress, is all about stress, a frequently overlooked but critical factor in gaining and losing fat—especially belly fat. First, you'll learn how to begin to know exactly what stress is and what it does to your body. Then we'll help you identify and defuse your own personal stressors. You'll learn three fantastically effective stress-busting practices from the science of mind-body medicine. You'll be able to start managing your stress better right away.

Part 4, Eating Away at Belly Fat, shows you that how you eat is almost as important as what you eat. You'll learn how to stop eating mindlessly and start savoring and enjoying your food. You'll see some fascinating research on the many reasons people eat that have nothing to do with hunger, and how to become a mindful eater. We'll also show you how to time your meals and snacks for optimal fat loss.

Part 5, On the Move, introduces you to a new way to move your body. We'll start by showing you smart ways to get more physical activity—just plain moving around—into each day. Then we'll share a lot of great and fun ideas for adding exercise to your life. You'll see that getting exercise doesn't have to be a chore. We'll show you exactly how much exercise you need and what types will be best for you.

Part 6, Getting Started, is where you get all the tools you need to get going. You'll do some self-assessments to see exactly where you are now, and learn how to track your progress as you move along toward that lean, flat belly. You'll learn how to start each day with a belly fat blast, and keep the fires burning all day with our delicious, easy-to-use recipes for breakfast, lunch, and snacks.

Part 7, Lean Belly Plan, picks up where Part 6 leaves off, taking you to the end of each day with recipes and ideas for dinners, salads, side dishes, and desserts. You'll also get a 14-day menu plan to get you off to a great, sure start. With all these recipes and menu plans, you won't have to wonder what to eat—and over time you'll be able to personalize your own flat belly plan that works best for you. More importantly, you'll learn how to make your new flat belly lifestyle permanent—so you'll never have to worry about belly fat again.

Extras

As you read our book, you'll find that it's peppered with lots of sidebars that contain juicy, concise content such as definitions, tips, warnings, and new research findings that will help you absorb and use the information in the book more quickly and easily.

DEFINITION

These sidebars provide you with definitions that are relevant to the topic at hand.

GOOD MOVE

Check these sidebars for tips to accelerate and maximize your belly fat loss.

RED FLAG

These sidebars describe common stumbling blocks that can prevent belly fat loss.

WHAT'S NEW

These sidebars tell you some of the latest, most exciting research on belly fat loss.

Acknowledgments

We'd like to thank two special women who were instrumental in getting this book written. Kate Patterson, ND, devoted hours of hard work to developing and writing most of the recipes in this book. As a board certified naturopathic physician trained in primary care, she believes that treating health (not disease) frees the body to return to a state of wellness naturally. Dr. Patterson received her training from the National College of Natural Medicine in Portland, Oregon, where she is now an adjunct faculty member. She's also in private practice at the Kenton Family Wellness Center in Portland.

Allie Purdy is a yoga teacher and yoga therapist as well as a mind-body medicine practitioner currently working in Portland, Oregon. She designed the yoga and core workout routines in this book. She is also the model for the photographs, demonstrating excellent form and technique. Her teaching schedule and bio are available at www.atuneyoga.com.

We'd like to extend effusive thanks to our editors, Brook Farling and Jennifer Bowles, who were patient beyond our wildest dreams as we worked our way through the early drafts of this book. They're consummate professionals and a joy to work with.

Marilyn Allen of the Allen O'Shea Literary Agency was our biggest cheerleader, and we will always be grateful to her for helping us get the opportunity to write this book.

Claire would like to thank her husband, Tim and her children, Eli, Walker, and Jackson for being so supportive and positive about the project.

Diane would like to thank her chef–computer guy husband Kevin for all the hard work and time he spent answering questions and running the household while Diane worked.

Special Thanks to the Technical Reviewer

The Complete Idiot's Guide to Belly Fat Weight Loss was reviewed by an expert who double-checked the accuracy of what you'll learn here, to help us ensure that this book gives you everything you need to know about belly fat weight loss. Special thanks are extended to Elizabeth DeRobertis, MS, RD, CDN, CDE.

Trademarks

All terms mentioned in this book that are known to be or are suspected of being trademarks or service marks have been appropriately capitalized. Alpha Books and Penguin Group (USA) Inc. cannot attest to the accuracy of this information. Use of a term in this book should not be regarded as affecting the validity of any trademark or service mark.

The Belly Fat Issue

Many people fret about the extra weight around their middle and with good reason. More than 60 percent of adult Americans are overweight or obese and most of this weight accumulates around our waists. Eating more junk food and drinking sugary beverages is certainly part of the problem, but it isn't the only reason belly fat is growing. It's also a result of the way we eat, the way we live, our genetic disposition, and high stress levels. As you'll see in this part, stress in particular plays a huge role in belly fat and disease. Each of these factors is discussed as well as why belly fat is worse for your health than the fat that accumulates in your legs or butt.

The myths surrounding belly fat are also dispelled, such as the idea that you have to be overweight to have it (you don't). Different ways are given to measure your own middle.

Getting Fat in the Modern World

In This Chapter

- The modern world is making us fat
- Bad fats and sugars are everywhere
- All day sitting can be toxic
- Stress makes it all worse

It's no secret that overweight and obesity rates in children, teenagers, and adults are increasing every year. In 2010, only about 29 percent of all American adults were at a healthy weight. Everyone else was either overweight or obese. What's really shocking about this explosion of obesity is that it happened so fast. In 1960, only about 14 percent of American adults were obese. Since then, that percentage has gone up to about 40 percent. Interestingly, the percentage of the population that is overweight but not obese has held pretty steady at around 32 percent.

This dramatic increase in the weight of the average person has brought with it a surge in the number of people with Type 2 diabetes, heart disease, and some types of cancer. Indeed, chronic disease is becoming the scourge of our time. Heart disease is the number one cause of death in both men and women, and the number of cases in the United States is expected to double in the next 50 years, as the current generation of overweight and obese children grows to adulthood.

How did this happen? What changed? Well, it certainly wasn't our DNA. What changed was our environment and our behavior, and even our ideas about what's normal when it comes to food, exercise, and stress. Before we get down to getting rid of belly fat, let's take a look at the reasons why so many of us are struggling to achieve and maintain good health.

Modern Lifestyles, Bulging Bellies

As you'll see, losing weight and avoiding obesity is not a simple matter of counting the calories you eat and doing a prescribed amount of exercise to burn them off. If it were that simple, the millions of people who start diet and exercise plans every year in the United States would be thin by now. It's well known by most health-care professionals that diets simply don't work. Unfortunately, it's been a tradition to simply blame the person who is struggling to be at a healthy weight for a lack of willpower or persistence. Even worse, it's commonly assumed that overweight people are too lazy to exercise.

WHAT'S NEW

Whether a person is overweight and/or obese is traditionally defined by the Body Mass Index (BMI), a calculation of the ratio between weight and height. When using pounds and inches, the BMI is equal to your weight in pounds times 703, divided by your height in inches squared (BMI = weight [in lbs] × 703, divided by height^2 [in inches]). There are many BMI calculators available online—refer to Appendix B to find some links. A person with a BMI of 25 or higher is overweight. A person with a BMI of 30 or higher is obese.

The most common way people try to lose weight is through a drastic reduction in calorie intake—to anywhere between 800 to 1,200 calories per day. Unfortunately, although this type of "dieting" can result in weight loss at first, it is almost never maintained. Not only do restrictive diets rarely lead to long-term weight loss—they can also be bad for your health because they can trigger an increase in stress hormone levels. Also, some research has shown that losing weight by dieting without exercise can lead to elevations in blood markers of inflammation.

This simplistic, somewhat moralistic approach to weight only makes the situation worse, adding shame and stigma to the other stresses that overweight and obese people have to deal with. The truth is that human beings are programmed to be world-class survivors of famine and food shortage. Until about 1,000 years ago, that's what all humans on the planet faced on a regular basis. In the Paleolithic world, being a survivor required the ability and drive to seek out food, eat a lot when food was available, and store extra calories as fat. These same tendencies lead to obesity, belly fat, and chronic disease in the modern world.

What we've done, with our drive-thru restaurants, automobiles, televisions, sedentary jobs, and high volume food production strategies, is create an environment in which human beings are entirely unsuited to thrive in. We have surrounded ourselves with just about every imaginable trigger to eat and a multitude of ways to avoid physical exertion. This may be pleasant and convenient for our modern minds, but it's absolutely toxic for our stone-age bodies.

Our Heritage: The Hunter-Gatherer

It's a fundamental principle of biology that living things thrive best in the environmental conditions they adapted to through thousands of years of natural selection. We human beings lived as hunter-gatherers for about 95 percent of our history on Earth, surviving by gathering plant foods and hunting animals for food. People tended to live in small bands that had to be somewhat nomadic, moving with changes in the seasons and weather, and the migration patterns of the animals they hunted.

GOOD MOVE

All of the dietary, activity, and stress management advice in this book is based on our understanding of the hunter-gatherer lifestyle—the environment our bodies are made to live in. Hunter-gatherers, also known as Paleolithic humans, lived simple lives that were centered around almost constant low to moderate levels of physical activity and a high-fiber plant-based diet. So whenever you're in doubt about how best to keep your belly fat burning, just remember, you can't go wrong by taking a walk or eating whole, unprocessed food.

For most of each year, hunter-gatherers could find adequate food to maintain health and vitality. In almost every climate, however, a few weeks or months of each year brought a season of food scarcity, or famine. Human beings adapted to this challenge by eating heartily when food was available and storing any extra energy in the form of fat. This stored energy would inevitably be used during the next season of food shortage.

The hunter-gatherer lifestyle required daily physical activity by every member of the community or tribe to acquire food. This physical activity was not especially intense, but it was consistent and varied. It's estimated that acquiring food required between 5 to 10 miles of walking or running every day. In addition, all labor was manual, requiring reaching, lifting, and carrying. In modern terms, this is a full day of aerobic, resistance, and flexibility exercises. Interestingly, the physical activity daily schedule of the hunter-gatherer was almost identical to the exercise regimens that are the most effective in preventing heart disease in this modern world.

The diet of the hunter-gatherer consisted entirely of what could be found or hunted. Archeologists estimate that about 75 to 80 percent of the total calories consumed came from the plant products they gathered, with the rest coming from animal sources. As the millennia passed, humans adapted the tendency to thrive on this balance of nutrients. Unfortunately, what the average person eats in this modern world is nothing like the food eaten by our genetically identical ancestors. It's estimated that about one-third of the calories in the standard American diet come from animal sources, and about half of that is eaten in the form of meat. This shift toward animal products and away from plants has led to big drops in our fiber and phytonutrient intake along with large increases in our consumption of saturated fat and cholesterol.

The Meaning of Meal Time

Another important thing about our hunter-gatherer ancestors is that they lived in highly interdependent, communal groups. This meant that social ties were not a source of amusement or companionship, but absolutely necessary for survival. As a result, we in the modern world are still hard-wired to seek companionship and supportive social networks.

Meal times especially were a time for social interaction. Unfortunately today, this very important part of traditional ways of eating is frequently overlooked. Family meals are on the decline, as fewer and fewer people eat at home, and more meals than ever are eaten on the run. These stressful and rushed ways of eating are in extreme contrast to the leisurely meals enjoyed with family and friends in the past.

RED FLAG

If you rarely sit down to eat a nice meal with your family, not only are you missing out on sharing vital socializing time with loved ones, you're losing out on the benefits of eating slowly and attentively.

Food, Stress, and Physical Inactivity

The lifestyle of the modern human being has almost nothing in common with the lifestyle our species "grew up" on. Our diet is nothing like what hunter-gatherers ate. We expend little or no physical effort to get our food—or to do anything for that matter. We have lost the essence of strong socially connected communal living and we are bombarded daily with stimuli and information that cause us worry, confusion, fear, or simply just sensory overload.

WHAT'S NEW

Noise, defined as "unwanted sound," has become a major part of the modern-day environment. Compared to the almost perfect silence enjoyed by our ancestors, we are subject to constant aural stimulation from television, sirens, motors, leaf blowers, traffic, and more. Recent research looking at the impact of our noisy world has yielded disturbing information. As your environment gets noisier, there is greater risk of insomnia, immune system suppression, and elevated stress hormones.

We have artificial lights that keep us up long after our bodies need to start sleeping. Our world is noisy, crowded, and contaminated with thousands of chemicals that are completely alien to our physiology. All in all, the hunter-gatherer inside each of us is living in a strange, hostile environment, and it's making us fat and sick.

The Way We Eat Today

The typical diet of the modern human being is drastically different from that eaten by Paleolithic man in almost every way, but research in dietary risk factors for heart disease has identified three changes that are particularly dangerous to our health:

1. We consume high quantities of manufactured fats such as *trans-fatty acids* instead of the plant-based unsaturated and polyunsaturated fats that are most supportive of health.

DEFINITION

Trans-fatty acids are vegetable fats that have been chemically altered to make them more stable at room temperature through a process called hydrogenation. This manufacturing process creates a fatty acid chain that is structurally differ-ent from all naturally occurring fatty acids. Trans fats were rapidly adopted by processed and packaged food manufacturers before it was discovered that they are dangerous to the heart and increase the risk of certain types of cancer.

2. We have seen an extreme increase in our consumption of omega-6 fatty acids, primarily from corn-fed beef and the corn and soybean oil used in processed foods. In contrast, we tend to consume many fewer omega-3 fatty acids, most of which come from fish, plants, and nuts.

3. The type and quantity of carbohydrates we eat now is nothing like what our ancestors consumed. The modern diet is extremely low in fiber, and appallingly high in simple sugars—this in contrast to the very high fiber, low sugar diet of the Paleolithic human.

Our bodies are designed to digest and absorb an optimal amount of each of the three macronutrients in food: protein, carbohydrates, and fat. The types and amounts of these macronutrients that have been found to be most beneficial to health in modern day are almost exactly the same as those found in the Paleolithic and Mediterranean diets. Protein should come from both plants and animals, and most people don't get enough in their diets. Animal protein should be lean, with an optimal ratio of omega-3 to omega-6 fatty acids—similar to that found in fatty fish such as salmon and lean cuts of grass-fed beef.

Bad Fats and Sugars

In the past few hundred years, the human diet has gone from being almost completely sugar free to being laden with sweeteners. Sweeteners make food more appealing and encourages consumption, so adding a little bit (even if you can't detect it, like in the case of ketchup) can significantly increase the amount a person will eat—and buy.

Sugar and *high fructose corn syrup (HFCS)* are the two most frequently used sweeteners in the modern diet. Cane sugar is a relatively natural substance, albeit highly refined and devoid of any nutritional value, and HFCS is a substance manufactured from corn. HFCS is extremely cheap compared to cane sugar, so it is much more widely used. The American diet is so saturated with HFCS that it's estimated that the average person in the United States consumes about 44 pounds of it every year.

DEFINITION

Invented in the 1970s, **high fructose corn syrup (HFCS)** is a sweetener manufactured from corn that, like cane sugar, is composed of two simple sugars—glucose and sucrose. Because of its slightly higher fructose content, HFCS is sweeter than sugar. Although it's a "natural" food, it is manufactured and therefore not exactly what the human body was designed to digest, leading many health experts to suggest that it may be more harmful to the body than cane sugar. On top of that, a disturbing study done by the Institute for Agriculture and Trade Policy in 2009 found that almost half of the samples of HFCS they tested contained mercury, an extremely toxic heavy metal that is frequently a contaminant in manufactured products.

Interestingly enough, the American diet became inundated with trans-fatty acids both for the sake of preserving processed foods and in a misguided effort to lure people away from eating butter. Trans fats are vegetable fats that are chemically manipulated to make them more resistant to becoming rancid over time and with exposure to oxygen. They were first invented early in the twentieth century, when food chemists discovered a way to add hydrogen to vegetable oils that were liquid at room temperature. The first "partially hydrogenated fat" made available to consumers was Crisco. During the Second World War, butter and other dairy products were rationed, so household cooks started using margarine and shortening instead.

In the late 1950s, the American Heart Association issued strong recommendations that people reduce the amount of saturated fats (found in meats; full-fat dairy products; and palm, palm kernel, and coconut oils) in their diets to avoid getting heart disease and replace them with trans fat products. This recommendation was based on very poor science and a hasty leap of logic that turned out to be incorrect—that these manufactured fats would be less harmful, and in fact beneficial to the people who ate them. The food and restaurant industries, on their own initiative and in response to huge consumer demand, gradually replaced most tropical and animal fats in the food they were producing.

By the early 1990s, several long-term studies of the connections between diet and heart disease, such as the Framingham Heart Study, began to document higher rates of heart disease in people who ate large amounts of trans-fatty acids. These people also had higher than usual levels of LDL (low-density lipoprotein) cholesterol, which is a strong risk factor for heart disease. These studies uncovered evidence that the liver, which is primarily responsible for metabolizing dietary fats and packaging them for delivery throughout the body, tends to make more LDL when trans fats are high in the diet. Elevated LDL is a strong risk factor for the development of coronary artery disease.

WHAT'S NEW

Many people have the mistaken idea that dietary cholesterol has a big impact on one's blood cholesterol levels. Not true. Dietary cholesterol has a much smaller impact on serum cholesterol when compared to the damage done by eating too many of the wrong types of fat, such as trans-fatty acids and some saturated fats.

In 2002, the U.S. government issued an official recommendation that people avoid eating trans fats, and in 2006, trans fat labeling on food packaging became mandatory. Consumers moved away from trans fats in droves, and thus ended a 40-year experiment in mass consumption of molecules that don't appear in nature and were never part of human nutrition.

Big Plates, Big Bellies

Since 1977, Americans have added an average of 300 calories (or 12 percent) per day to their diets. During this same time period, there's been no change in the average amount of physical activity that we engage in every day. Three hundred extra calories a day may not seem like a lot, but over months and years, it amounts to a large excess of energy being taken in. Because these calories aren't being burned, they have to be stored as fat.

Studies of human eating behavior have uncovered several triggers for overeating that many people aren't aware of. One major cue to eat more is simply to have more food put in front of you. This is exactly what's happened here in the United States and abroad—serving sizes of food and beverages have grown steadily bigger since the late 1970s. If you're older than 40, you probably remember a time when there was no such thing as a Big Gulp soft drink and the Big Mac hadn't appeared at McDonald's.

The United States Department of Agriculture (USDA) has long taken responsibility for prescribing the amount of all kinds of food Americans should eat each day. Although these recommendations have remained fairly stable, the actual portion sizes offered in packaged food and in restaurants have ballooned drastically. The biggest portion increases have occurred in cookies, which are now a staggering seven times as large as they were in 1980. Pasta servings are now almost five times their previous size and steaks have doubled.

RED FLAG

The more meals you eat each week away from home, the more likely it is that you're consuming too many calories and too many unhealthy additives such as bad fats and sweeteners. Even stopping at a coffee shop each morning instead of taking a go-cup from home can be a bad idea, as it's hard to resist the pastry display every morning.

There are some interesting reasons for this apparent generosity among food manufacturers and restaurants. First of all, a basic principle of doing business is making customers happy. People feel like they're getting a deal when they get a lot more food for a little more money, and this builds brand loyalty. In addition, our basic hunter-gatherer appetite revels in quantity, so bigger servings are an easy sell. The profit margins on prepared and processed foods are so great—on average about 80 percent—that companies can easily afford to give you more food to ensure that you'll keep coming back to buy what they're offering.

While all this was going on in the last couple decades, another big shift in our eating behavior was happening that made the situation even worse. Americans steadily increased the number of meals eaten away from home. This is probably because we've had a big increase in the number of two-income families, longer commutes, and longer work hours. Many people just feel too tired and stressed out to cook at the end of a long day. In 1977, the percentage of food the average American kid ate away from home was about 6.5 percent. Now it's nearly tripled to about 19.3 percent.

As we drifted out into the world of fast food restaurants and convenience stores to feed ourselves, we gladly consumed more and more food, happy to be finding "bargains." After a while, expanded portion sizes started to seem normal—and people serve themselves too much food when they eat at home, too.

So now, when the average American reaches for a "serving" of salty snacks such as potato chips, she ends up eating 225 calories instead of 132 calories. The average serving of french fries in 1977 delivered about 188 calories—now it delivers 256. The average hamburger calories have risen from 389 to 486. Everywhere you go, you're tempted with the comfort of more food and the gratification of getting it for less money.

Unhealthy Food Is Everywhere

Larger serving sizes are not the only downside of taking your meals on the road. The quality of food eaten outside the home is almost always inferior to the nutritional value of home-cooked meals and snacks. This, too, is driven mostly by the restaurant's and manufacturer's goal to give customers as satisfying an eating experience as they can, because a happy, sated customer is one who will gladly return for more.

How do they do it? Giving us a lot of food is only the beginning. The food they give us is specifically and deliberately engineered to be more *palatable*. Foods become more palatable when they're high in fat and sweeteners—so restaurant and convenience foods are often packed with both. Of course, whenever you add fat and sugar to a food, you also increase the number of calories per bite.

DEFINITION

Palatability is the quality of food that makes it pleasant to eat. Highly palatable foods tend to be high in sucrose and/or saturated fats, but this can vary from person to person. Palatable food tends to trigger overeating and a shorter interval between one meal or snack and another because of an increased desire for food.

If we look at this manipulation of food from the perspective of the hunter-gatherer, this artificial palatability starts to appear less fun and benign. Sweet, fatty foods are delightful to our palate because our Paleolithic ancestors rarely came across this type of nourishment. A body that has to walk, sometimes miles for every meal, is going to ravenously consume the occasional treasure of a sweet morsel that has fat added. It just makes sense in the economy of calories in and out. So we have evolved to love sweet, fatty foods, not because they objectively have better flavor than other foods, but because there's a survival advantage to liking them when you need to get as many calories per bite as possible in the face of cyclical famine.

Palatability affects our appetite in many ways. Because it confers an ancient (but no longer necessary) survival advantage, palatable food triggers significant changes in the brain such as release of endorphins that have a calming and euphoric effect. Palatability stimulates you to eat more than you normally would for any given meal or snack—but its effects don't end when you're done eating. Highly palatable food may cause a faster, steeper increase in blood sugar than an equal amount of less palatable food, especially if it contains sugar or white flour. This spike in blood sugar tends to lead to a quicker return of hunger after eating. So you go back and get more of that food that was so delicious—and the company that sold it to you is only too happy to sell you more!

Sitting Still

While all this expansion of our food intake has been going on, the physical activity levels of adults have stayed pretty much the same. Worse yet, children appear to be getting less and less exercise. With the closing of physical education programs in schools and recreation programs in municipal and city parks, kids just have fewer opportunities for organized physical activity. Kids are much more likely to get out and exercise if they're in a class or a program than on their own initiative. This is because, for most kids, it's more fun to watch television or play video games than it is to play outside.

Adults are also more likely to opt for convenience and comfort instead of physical effort. This, again, is just part of our hunter-gatherer physiology. We're designed to take in all available energy and spend as little energy as possible to get those calories, because we're designed to withstand famine and starvation. It's not laziness, it's an ancient drive for energy conservation.

WHAT'S NEW

Inactivity physiology is the term that describes the newly recognized and drastic changes that occur in the human body when it's sedentary. It turns out that being sedentary isn't just bad for you because you're missing out on the benefits of exercise—it's actually toxic. So far, studies have shown that people who sit more than 6 hours a day have alarming and dangerous changes in their physiology such as large drops in HDL (the good cholesterol) and large increases in blood sugar (a setup for diabetes).

Clever animals that we are, we've come up with dozens, perhaps hundreds of ways to minimize the physical effort required to get through an ordinary day. Exercise physiologists are only recently beginning to discover and document the many consequences of not moving like a hunter-gatherer every day. It's becoming quite clear that avoiding belly fat and overall weight gain is almost impossible if you don't use your skeletal muscles enough to stimulate them to help burn energy and absorb blood sugar from the food you eat each day.

Cars, Elevators, and Drive-Thrus

If you spent a day noting every time you chose a physically easier way to do just about anything, you'd find that it's a habitual tendency, one you may not even notice while you're doing it. Without thinking, we choose the escalator instead of the stairs, the drive-thru teller instead of going into the bank, and the automatic walkway at the airport instead of simply walking. If the convenience is there, people will use it.

Since 1977, the percentage of errands and outings taken by adults on foot have decreased about 40 percent while we've increased our use of cars by 90 percent. Now, this is due in part because many of us live in suburban or rural areas that lack walking-distance access to work, the grocery store, etc. But even when these things are only a short walk away, most people choose to drive. It's become normal to drive even very short distances to accomplish our necessary activities and errands.

The Scourge of Screens

A recent survey of American children between the ages of 8 and 18 years old found that the average kid spends about 6 hours a day in front of screens. The kids in this study accumulated this screen time by watching an average of 4 hours of television, playing about an hour of video games, and spending another hour using a computer every day. This was after a full day of school.

Adults are also prone to choosing the screen over physical activity. Several studies have shown that the number of hours spent watching television per week is directly associated with weight and BMI. Worse yet, as television time increases, so does the risk of developing diabetes and heart disease. TV time has a big impact on your weight for a couple of reasons. First of all, you're being completely sedentary while you're doing it. Secondly, people are much more likely to snack while watching television than when engaged in any other activity (if you can call watching TV an activity).

GOOD MOVE

The latest trend among fitness and weight experts is the standing desk—a desk that's high enough to allow you to do all your work while standing. This one move can help you burn many more calories per day and keep your blood sugar and cholesterol down.

The average American adult spends almost 5 hours a day watching television, which amounts to about 9 solid years of TV in a lifetime. About 66 percent of Americans routinely watch TV while eating dinner. When asked, half of all American adults say they watch too much television. Many people spend an additional 2 or 3 hours a day at their home computers, surfing the internet, watching media, and playing games. This amounts to a second full-time job—one spent entirely sedentary and usually isolated from social interaction, which is a critical factor in protecting people from the bad health effects of stress.

The Stress Factor

Stress is a psychological, emotional, and physical state that arises whenever you feel threatened or overwhelmed by what's happening in your life. Your body's stress reaction is the product of thousands of years of human life spent in a very primitive setting that was fraught with frequent threats to safety and survival. While our stress physiology hasn't changed, the world we live in is totally different, presenting, for most people, lots of stressors but very few actual life-threatening events. So here we are in the twenty-first century, under pressure from our jobs, money woes, social obligations, family responsibilities, having too much to do, and more.

More than half of the people surveyed reported that stress was making them feel frequently angry or irritable, fatigued, and unable to sleep at night. In Chapter 3, we'll take a look at the pathway from stressful thoughts and events through weight gain to increased risk of illness and even premature death.

Information Overload

Of all the stress triggers people are exposed to, the most difficult to manage are those we have no control over. Before the era of mass communication, humans mostly dealt with immediate, tangible problems that could at least be addressed, if not solved, by taking some sort of action. Nowadays, people are bombarded with all kinds of distressing information, a lot of which has no direct effect on us at all, that we can't do anything about.

Floods, war, pollution, global warming, terrorism—it's all on the news every day, presented with an air of urgency that's hard to resist. Every evening during regular television, we're teased with promotions for that night's late news stories, usually with fear-based messages such as, "Is your cell phone giving you brain cancer? Story at 11!"

 RED FLAG

Many people make it a habit to watch the late news before going to bed, and this can be a bad idea. Taking in all the world's troubles can create a stress reaction that in turn can make it hard to get a good night's sleep. If you're a nighttime news junkie, consider holding off until morning, and listening to some soothing music or doing some light reading before lights out.

Even the things we could control are often coming at us so quickly that it's hard to keep up. Kids' schedules, parents' needs, budgets, bills, even our entertainment and communication gadgets all provide a constant source of stimulation and distraction from our thoughts and feelings. The solution isn't to hide away in a cave somewhere but to start paying attention to how all this stimulation makes you feel, and to start weeding out the overwhelming, uncontrollable stressors from the things in life you can control and really care about. We'll look at ways to do this in later chapters on stress management.

Worries, Worries, Worries

Stress is a growing problem for people all over the world. In 2008, the American Psychological Association conducted a nationwide poll on the status of stress in the everyday life of American adults. What they found is sobering. Half of the respondents reported that their stress levels have increased during the past year, and 30 percent rated their stress levels as "extreme." Eighty percent of people reporting high levels of stress attributed them to financial losses and uncertainty along with job insecurity or unemployment.

Half of all American adults feel stressed about being able to provide for their family's needs. Stress over money and job stability used to be more common in men, but with more women in the work force and a greater proportion of them being single mothers, provider stress has become slightly more prevalent in women than men.

While there will always be things to worry about and life will always challenge you, it's possible to protect yourself from the ravages of stress and worry. Good stress management isn't just good for your peace of mind—it's good for your belly, because stress is one of the biggest reasons why people put on belly fat. We'll look at just how that happens in Chapter 3.

The Least You Need to Know

- The first step in getting rid of belly fat is to recognize that your body was built to thrive on simple, whole food, not fake fats and sugars.
- Modern food manufacturing has brought us a deluge of highly palatable food in even bigger serving sizes, available everywhere, leading to an average of 300 extra calories per day for the average person.
- Sitting down for 6 or more hours a day is considered part of the normal American lifestyle—and it's a major risk factor for belly fat and heart disease.
- Stress feeds belly fat, so you're going to need to recognize the stressors in your life and learn effective ways to cope with them to defuse stress's ability to bloat your belly.

What's Belly Fat?

In This Chapter

- What belly fat is and why it matters so much
- How belly fat can threaten your health
- What the best ways are to measure belly and body fat
- How to debunk belly fat myths

The "inch you can pinch" is the layer of subcutaneous (below the skin) fat you can grab at your middle. Although subcutaneous fat is an indication of overall overweight and obesity, it isn't the fat that we call "belly fat."

Belly fat goes by several different names, including mesenteric fat, intra-abdominal fat, and visceral fat. What all of these terms are referring to is a unique type of fat tissue that collects inside your abdomen. This type of fat differs from subcutaneous fat (the fat that collects under your skin) in many critical ways that we'll examine in this chapter.

We'll also look at how you can best figure out how much fat is on your body right now, and how much of that fat is inside your belly. There are a few different ways to do this, but as you'll see, the simplest way is with your scale and a tape measure. Finally, we'll debunk a few widely held myths about belly fat and how it comes and goes.

Belly Fat Is Unique

Belly fat is made by your body as part of your overall stress response. It is created when cortisol levels are high. Cortisol is the primary steroid of stress that our bodies make to help us respond to stressful situations that are long-lasting, or chronic.

For hunter-gatherers, the most common type of chronic stress was famine, whether that occurred during the course of a long, cold winter or other conditions when food was scarce. During those times, the body has to be prepared for the daily struggle to find food and carry out all the other essential tasks of life. During this chronic stress, whenever the Paleolithic human found something to eat, he ate as much as he could, sometimes consuming a few more calories than he needed right at that moment.

Whenever you take in more calories than you need, your body has to figure out what to do with the extra energy you've taken in. Because we're built to expect food shortages at any time, our bodies are designed to store this energy instead of burning it off. Depending on your stress levels, you'll store extra calories as fat in one of two places.

RED FLAG

It doesn't take much in the way of extra eating and drinking or too little exercise to pack on the fat. Getting just 100 calories a day more than what you need can amount to a 10-pound weight gain in the course of a year. Stress and a comfort-food rich diet can make your body even more likely to store those extra calories as fat.

Think of a house with a garage and an attic. Holiday decorations, baby clothes, old yearbooks, and other things that aren't needed often tend to be put away in the attic, sometimes for years at a time. Bicycles, raingear, and gardening tools tend to be stored in the garage for quick and easy access. You can think of the fat deposits that lie just under the skin on the hips, thighs, breasts, and other parts of the body as your body's fat attic. Fat is stored there in times of low stress, when there's no apparent need for a quick burst of energy and power to meet a crisis.

Sticking with the house metaphor, think of belly fat as the garage. When you gain weight during stressful times, your body chooses to store extra energy in the belly, because the fat stored there can be easily broken down into triglycerides and other forms of fat that can travel through the bloodstream to provide energy to other tissues and organs. As the amount of fat in your belly increases, so may the level of triglycerides in your blood, because your belly fat is doing its job of keeping these levels elevated in preparation for the impending life-or-death struggle that never happens.

It's Internal

Belly fat collects inside the abdomen. Most of it is deposited on two major intra-abdominal structures—the mesentery and the omentum. The mesentery is a fibrous structure that is attached to the back of the abdominal wall. It's made up of sheaths of tissue that hold the intestines and other abdominal organs in place inside the belly. The omentum is like an apron of fibrous tissue that hangs down between the abdominal organs and the abdominal wall, offering protection against pressure and blows to the belly. Normally, these two structures have very little fat on them.

GOOD MOVE

Belly fat goes by many different names that all refer to the same thing—a collection of fat cells inside the abdomen. It is much more hazardous to your health than the readily visible subcutaneous fat most people worry about. These cells not only store fat, but also attract inflammatory cells of the immune system, and congregate to form what's essentially a new body organ—one that makes stress worse and secretes dozens of molecules that can endanger health over time.

Belly fat can also collect around the organs themselves. Over time, as these fat stores enlarge, they increase the circumference of your torso, especially at the waistline, creating that "apple" shape associated with abdominal overweight and obesity.

It's Not Just for Storage

Belly fat can be thought of as an endocrine organ in its own right—that is, an organ that secretes chemicals into the bloodstream that elicit significant changes in the activity of other organs. So far, researchers have found dozens of chemicals that belly fat releases, and there are most likely many more yet to be discovered.

Belly fat cells produce and secrete several types of immune system stimulants called cytokines. These molecules circulate around the body revving up certain cells of immunity that are in charge of inflammation. These cells are only supposed to be fired up in the face of an injury or extreme physical stress. They promote wound healing and blood clotting, among other things. When these cells, most of which are known as macrophages, stay on red alert for long periods of time, they can get involved in the formation of arterial plaque, which bulges into the arteries of your heart, brain, and other areas and leads to heart attack and stroke. We'll look further into the risks of inflammation later in this chapter and in Chapter 3.

One of the most important chemicals released by abdominal fat cells is resistin. Resistin is a chemical that acts on insulin receptors on cells throughout the body to make them resist the effect of insulin. This makes sense when you think of what the human body needs in a long-term crisis—more fat and sugar to keep going. If this goes on for years, however, it can develop into one of the most dangerous chronic conditions of the modern world—Type 2 Diabetes Mellitus. As we go along you'll see how belly fat, poor diet, and insulin resistance can work together to drastically increase your risk of diabetes, heart disease, stroke, and dying before your time.

The Dangers of Too Much Belly Fat

Belly fat exists to keep your body primed for an imminent life-threatening crisis—so it's all about keeping fuel available and your acute stress response simmering. There are four primary ways that belly fat threatens your health, and they all have to do with belly fat's role as part of your overall response to chronic stress. Belly fat causes:

- Elevated blood levels of fat and cholesterol
- Chronic elevations in blood sugar and insulin
- Persistent low-level inflammation
- Amplified stress responses

When you put all these effects together, they can be life-saving if you're truly in a famine or other long-term challenge to your physical well-being. But in the presence of plentiful amounts of high-calorie, high-fat, high-sugar palatable food, these effects are life-threatening.

Elevated Fat and Cholesterol in the Blood

As you've seen, belly fat is stored in such a way that it can be rapidly broken down for use by the rest of the body. When belly fat is present, blood triglyceride levels may remain chronically elevated. This elevation in blood triglycerides sends a message to the liver that the body is stressed and needs more fat and cholesterol.

The liver is in charge of processing everything you eat and packaging the energy (especially the fats) in exactly the way the body needs it. When the liver is receiving a signal that the body needs lots of energy, it tends to make and release more cholesterol in the LDL form. LDL cholesterol, also known as the "bad" cholesterol, has a high fat content, which makes it a potent source of energy, but also makes it more vulnerable to oxidation.

GOOD MOVE

Antioxidants are chemicals found in plants such as fruits, vegetables, coffee, and red wine. These chemicals protect you against the damage done by stress and belly fat because they deactivate the dangerous by-products of metabolism, preventing oxidation of LDL and other fats. From the first day of this program, you'll be getting plenty of antioxidants and reaping this tremendous benefit.

All fats, whether they're inside your body or sitting in a jar on your kitchen counter, are vulnerable to becoming rancid. Fats become rancid after exposure to oxygen. Oxygen molecules interact with the molecular structure of fat cells to change their shape, which can make them smell bad, and make them potentially harmful to the human body.

LDL cholesterol collects in arterial walls and other tissues of the body to provide energy, but when there's too much of it, the oxygen in the blood can react with it to make it rancid. When that happens, the fat is potentially harmful, and now a target for the cells of the immune system. As you'll see, arterial plaque (atherosclerosis) is the cause of heart attacks and strokes, and plaque is formed when immune cells in the arteries attack and engulf oxidized LDL.

Elevated Blood Sugar and Insulin Resistance

The cells of the body that require insulin in order to take up sugar are the skeletal muscles and fat cells. Brain cells do not need insulin to be able to take up sugar. The brain has to be the body's first priority for energy allocation—because if your brain stops working, you can't function at all. So insulin regulation of blood sugar uptake by other cells serves to make sure that the brain always has first dibs on whatever sugar is available—even when food is very scarce.

WHAT'S NEW

Being overweight or obese is a major precursor to Type 2 diabetes, but new research shows that it's belly fat in particular, not overall fatness, that is the biggest danger. It's been found that waist circumference (a measure of belly fat) is a much better predictor of a person's diabetes risk than the BMI, which only looks at weight, presumably because of belly fat's impact on blood sugar and insulin receptors.

When insulin receptors aren't responding properly to insulin's signals, the sugar isn't being allowed into the cells. The net effect of this is that blood sugar remains high. If food is scarce, this is great. If food is plentiful, this is a real problem, because eating a lot of food generates a lot of blood sugar that isn't being controlled properly by insulin.

What we call blood sugar is actually known as glucose in the body. Glucose is absolutely essential to life—but when its levels get too high, it can be a toxin. It causes damage to the delicate cells that line blood vessels and the delicate nerve endings found in the skin of the extremities. Over time, this damage leads to atherosclerosis in the heart and brain (which causes heart attacks and strokes) and impaired sensation in the toes and feet (which leads to the repeated injury and damage that necessitates amputations in people with diabetes).

Increased General Inflammation

Belly fat, unlike peripheral fat, attracts macrophages, the cells of the immune system that are involved in creating inflammation. It's not clear why, but over time, belly fat becomes a beehive of activated macrophages that continually make and release into the bloodstream a set of chemicals called pro-inflammatory cytokines. What these chemicals are designed to do is recruit and activate immune cells from all over the body to assist in some kind of acute or ongoing infection or tissue damage.

It appears that a slightly elevated level of body-wide inflammation is part of the stress response. When you consider that ancient stressors frequently involved being injured in a fight or sustaining tissue damage while fleeing or hunting for food, it makes sense that the part of the immune system that specializes in immediate responses to injury would be put on high alert. And this is exactly what happens.

Unfortunately, this situation was never meant to go on for months, years, and decades. But the stressors of modern life do go on that long, and in the absence of a healthy diet, good stress management, and frequent physical activity, so does the smoldering fire of chronic stress and inflammation.

Chronic low-level inflammation is a strong risk factor for coronary artery disease. This is especially so when LDL levels are high. Here's what happens—LDL is not inherently bad. In fact it's a beautifully constructed package made by the liver out of protein molecules, cholesterol, and fatty acids for the purpose of delivering the energy contained in the fats to the cells of the body. In the well-fed, unstressed person, LDL levels tend to stay within healthy limits and do their job—feed all the cells, tissues, and structures that make up the human body.

The arteries are among those structures that use the energy packed in LDLs to nourish their cells. LDL travels through the bloodstream and can readily enter the walls of arteries where it normally would quickly fall apart, releasing its fuel right where it's needed. But in the stressed, poorly fed, and under-exercised body, things don't go the way they should.

Belly Fat Makes Stress Worse

As you'll see in the next chapter, cortisol is the major hormone of stress. It promotes overeating, fat storage, belly fat, and a variety of potentially unhealthy changes when it's elevated over time. Every person's blood has cortisol present in both an inactive and an active form. The hormone becomes active when changed by a specific enzyme that is located in fat tissue.

This cortisol-activating enzyme is much more plentiful in abdominal fat than subcutaneous fat. As belly fat grows, so does the number of these enzymes and so does the blood levels of cortisol, which only perpetuates stress and makes it worse. Belly fat elevates cortisol, which in turn triggers a more voracious appetite, craving for sugar and fat, and weight gain. This vicious cycle is very hard to break without paying attention not only to food and exercise, but stress levels.

How to Measure Body and Belly Fat

Having too much fat on and in your body, as we've seen, can put you at higher risk of heart disease, diabetes, and other medical problems. But the issue isn't just fat. The ratio of fat to muscle and bone is also important, especially for regulating blood sugar. According to the American Council on Exercise, the ideal amount of fat as a percentage of your total body weight is between 21 to 33 percent for women and 14 to 24 percent for men.

Traditionally, the health risks of fat have been predicted using a person's weight, or the Body Mass Index (BMI), a ratio between weight and height. Although this ratio has been useful for tracking long-term changes in large populations, it's not ideal for assessing any one person's risks associated with fat or belly fat.

What's Wrong with the BMI

The Body Mass Index (BMI) has been the international standard for determining whether a person is overweight or obese since the 1980s. It's a mathematical ratio between your weight and your height squared, times a constant. A person's BMI increases as weight goes up for a given height, so higher BMIs correspond with overweight and obesity.

Based on large observational studies of the correlations between BMI and health outcomes, a set of standards was established for what constitutes being overweight, or being obese. A "normal weight" was determined by identifying people with the lowest risk of fat-associated diseases. "Overweight" was the classification given to people with an increased risk of these health problems, and "obesity" is the classification for people at high risk. The condition of obesity has three classes. People with Class I obesity have high risk, people with Class II obesity have very high risk, and those with Class III obesity are at extremely high risk of fat-related diseases.

This system works well for watching trends in large groups of people, because in any large population, especially in the developed world, weight gain occurs because of an increase in body fat. The BMI isn't always the best way to assess any given individual's risk, however, because it gives no indication of two critical factors—body composition and fat distribution.

For example, if you calculated the BMI of two men, both of whom were 6 feet tall and weighed 265 pounds, you'd come up with 37.3 and classify them both with Class II obesity, at a very high risk of disease. But if one of the men was a football player, with only 12 percent body fat and minimal belly fat—you'd be wrong! This is a problem, but it's pretty easy to tell an obese man from a football player.

An even bigger, and potentially dangerous, problem with the BMI is that, at the lower end of the scale, it can't discern between a 70-year-old woman with a BMI of 20 because she's lean and strong and has little fat and another 70-year-old woman whose BMI is 20 because she has lost most of her muscle mass and bone density. Sadly, the latter situation is a common problem as people age.

There's no doubt that for most people younger than age 70, body weight and BMI are reasonable ways to determine fat-related health risks. But it's also become clear from the research that two people with the same BMI but very different waist sizes will also probably have very different risks to their health.

Measuring Body Fat

The gold standard for measuring your body fat content is underwater weighing. This can be costly and hard to find. With this technique, you are first weighed on a scale and then weighed fully immersed in water. The difference between your weight in air and your weight under water gives an indication of your body's density. Bone and muscle are denser than fat—so the less dense you are, the more fat you have on your body. With underwater weighing, you get the percentage of fat but no information about where that fat is being stored—so it's not great for figuring out how much belly fat you have.

There are other more convenient and affordable ways to estimate body fat. Some doctors and athletic trainers use skin calipers to estimate body fat percentage. This technique can be accurate to within 5 percentage points, but it has to be done carefully, by someone experienced.

WHAT'S NEW

DEXA scanning is a special technique based on low-dose x-rays that measures body density. It can determine the difference between lean and fat body mass, as well as the location of body fat. Frequently used to measure bone density in women at risk of osteoporosis, this technique is an extremely reliable (but very expensive) way to assess body and belly fat.

It's also possible to buy a home scale that measures your weight and your body's density. It's hard to get a truly accurate measure of body fat with an at-home scale, but you can measure your progress—and that's what's important. If you decide to track your body fat percentage with an at-home scale, make sure you follow these tips:

- Use the calibration features on the scale, entering your sex and age.

- Measure your weight and body fat at the same time of day, ideally about an hour after drinking one cup of water. Drinking the water is a way to ensure that your fluid balance is fairly consistent from measurement to measurement.

- Don't measure yourself after exercise, because sweating sets off your fluid balance in unpredictable ways.

Whether or not you decide to measure and track your body composition, you must measure and track your weight and the circumferences of your waist and hips at the very beginning and once a week during the program.

Measuring Belly Fat

Estimating belly fat is relatively easy to do. All you need for a rough estimate is a tape measure. Whatever your weight, it's important to know how big around your waist is. While the plan in this book will help you lose weight, the more important goal will be to achieve a smaller waist, because that means you're getting rid of a major risk to your health—as well as improving your overall appearance and how you feel each day.

For women, waist circumference should be 35 inches or less, and for men, 40 inches or less. To measure your waist circumference, stand up straight and place your tape measure around your middle, at its narrowest, just above your hip bones. Take the measurement just after your breathe out—but don't strain to suck in your belly.

Consistency is key to tracking your progress. You should take your body measurements at the same time of day. The best time to do this is in the morning, after you've emptied your bladder but before you eat or drink anything. Make sure you measure the same part of your abdomen each time.

Common Myths About Belly Fat

Belly fat, as you've seen, is much more than a dormant wad of excess calories lodged inside your abdomen. It's a highly active, potentially dangerous organ that stress, poor diet, and lack of exercise work together to create. It's easy to identify some people with belly fat if they have the classic apple shape or beer belly. But what about people who aren't obviously overweight? Can they have belly fat?

Many people feel resigned to the idea that they're destined to have a big belly because it's a common and relatively normal part of aging. Not so. It's also a myth that belly fat is hard to lose and you may as well just live with it. This myth has been promoted by the widespread belief that you have to achieve some "ideal weight" in order to be healthier and feel better. Again—not true!

You Have to Be Overweight to Have It

Fat can collect in your belly even if you're not technically overweight or obese. A study was done recently to examine the effects of modest weight gain on healthy adults. Participants had their diets manipulated to take their BMI from an average of 23.1 to 24.6—still below the cutoff for "overweight." The people who gained the weight showed dramatic increases in their belly fat mass—and big changes in their blood levels of insulin, triglycerides, and cholesterol—all in the direction of greater risk for heart disease and other chronic disorders.

Other studies have shown that even lean people can have belly fat buildup, and this belly fat is just as metabolically active and dangerous as it is in the overweight and obese. If you're eating poorly, not getting enough exercise, and not managing stress well, you could be carrying belly fat even if you look thin.

In fact, there's a term for this—normal weight obesity, which is the term that refers to a person with a "healthy" weight and/or BMI but too high a percentage of body fat. More and more, we're finding out that focusing on weight isn't nearly as important as maintaining a healthy lifestyle and keeping your belly flat.

WHAT'S NEW

Normal weight obesity is an ever-increasingly common condition in the United States. Poor diet and a sedentary lifestyle lead to excess body fat, belly fat, and harmful changes in metabolism even in people who appear to be thin and maintain a healthy weight.

It's Hard to Get Rid Of

It may seem that there's nothing but bad news about belly fat, but here's some great news—it's the easiest kind of fat to get rid of. In fact, belly fat is the first to go in 99 percent of all people who start losing weight. That means that you will start reaping the health benefits of belly fat loss right from the start, and with every pound you lose.

This makes sense when you recall that belly fat is an emergency energy store, meant to be easily broken down in case of danger or food shortage. Starting on this program or any other that involves eating a little less and moving a little more takes your body out of energy storage mode and into energy burning. The quickest and easiest way for your body to do that is to start breaking down belly fat.

Knowing this, you can stop stressing about getting to a certain weight to be healthier. You can start this flat-belly program confident that from day one, your belly fat is melting away, and your waist is getting smaller.

It's a Normal Part of Aging

While the risk of belly fat goes up with age, that doesn't mean it's an inevitable part of getting older. Belly fat appears as stress levels go up and diets become poorer, but for the aging, it's probably most strongly linked to drops in physical activity for most adults, and to hormonal changes that come with menopause in women. It may be harder to keep belly fat at bay as you get older, but it's certainly not impossible if you stick to the lifestyle guidelines in this book.

Human growth hormone (HGH) is released in ever-decreasing amounts as many people age, and these lower levels of HGH are associated with belly fat buildup. For years, it was assumed that HGH levels fell naturally with aging. Recent research has shown that as long as you keep moving, your HGH levels won't fall as far as those in a sedentary person—and HGH helps keep your lean-to-fat body composition in a healthier range by supporting and maintaining skeletal muscle development. No matter how old you are, you're always eligible for a lean belly and active, vibrant body!

WHAT'S NEW

Osteoporosis, a condition in which the bones lose their mineral density and become easily broken, is a common condition among women as they age. In most studies, being overweight hasn't been found to be an important risk factor for osteoporosis. Recently, however, researchers have found a link between belly fat and bone density. It appears that in premenopausal women, as belly fat goes up, bone density tends to go down. It's not clear how belly fat causes bone loss, but keeping strong, healthy bones is another good reason to lose it.

The Least You Need to Know

- Belly fat is a particularly dangerous form of fat that collects inside your abdomen.
- Belly fat accumulation is a hard-wired part of the human stress response.
- Belly fat is associated with elevated LDL, triglycerides, and blood sugar, along with markers of chronic inflammation—all risk factors for a variety of diseases.
- Body composition and waist circumference are better measures of your health risks due to fat than your weight or BMI.
- Even lean, "healthy" weight people can have excess belly fat if they don't eat well and get enough exercise.

Stress, Belly Fat, and Disease

In This Chapter

- Stress increases belly fat in two important ways
- Stress is a whole-body response to your perceptions
- Cortisol is stress's belly fat producer
- Stress and belly fat work together to cause disease

The condition of your body when you're chronically stressed out is a perfect setup for overeating, gaining weight, and having most of that fat end up inside your belly. Belly fat is a unique kind of fat that functions more like a stress gland than a simple storage facility for excess calories.

Harmful stress is not the inevitable result of life's challenges, problems, losses, and disappointments. Life, for most people, presents challenges both big and small pretty much every day. The key to good stress management isn't to strive for a hassle-free life, but to learn how to put things into perspective, take an active role in tackling problems, and to learn effective ways to keep mind and body calm and clear in the face of stress.

We used to think that stress was only a problem for people going through life events such as divorce, unemployment, death of a spouse, and other big catastrophes. Although these conditions certainly lead to stress in many people, newer research has revealed that everyday hassles such as long commutes, marital dissatisfaction, job stress, and financial woes are just as likely to lead to the ravages of chronic stress. Whether it's a major life change or the little upsets of every day, life can be overwhelming at times, and that's where good stress management becomes vital to belly fat loss and good health.

Stress physiology leads to disease in several ways. The most important outcomes of chronic stress include:

- More body fat, especially belly fat
- High blood pressure and cardiovascular stress
- Elevated cholesterol, sugar, and insulin levels
- Greater risk of obesity, diabetes, and heart disease

This chapter looks at the nitty gritty of stress's impact on your behavior, mind, and body. You'll see how being a stressed-out person can make you more vulnerable to belly fat buildup, chronic disease, and even dying too soon.

Stress's Two-Pronged Attack

Stress piles on the pounds in two basic ways—by triggering coping behaviors that may make you feel better, but are generally bad for your health, and by creating a physical state that causes a lot of undue wear and tear on your system.

First of all, people under stress are more likely to have poor health habits than people who aren't bothered by stress.

Coping refers to the thoughts and behaviors you turn to when sensing that life is challenging and stressful. There are good (healthy) and bad (unhealthy) ways to cope with stress. Most people cope in ways that are learned—from parents, peers, and the media. There are two types of coping: Problem Management (taking active steps to solve problems) and Emotional Regulation (making use of specific skills and techniques to relieve negative emotions). In general, all types of stressors tend to trigger some type of emotional regulation, whether healthy—like exercise or talking with a friend—or less healthy—like drinking too much alcohol or eating junk food. Problem management is almost always a positive, healthy type of coping because it's all about changing the situation for the better.

DEFINITION

Coping is an individual's set of cognitive and behavioral responses to their perceptions of threat and challenge in everyday life. These threats can come from the world outside or from scary thoughts, ideas, or memories.

Stress is also a physical state of emergency. Our stress responses developed to make survival in the hunter-gatherer environment more likely—in the face of primitive stressors such as physical attacks from predators and other humans, prolonged lack of food, extremes of weather and climate, etc. Because the stress response involves extreme changes to most bodily functions, it's hazardous and wasteful when it's activated for long periods of time.

How Stress Changes Behavior

Most people turn to unhealthy, momentary pleasures when they're feeling a lot of pressure and stress. This is most likely because being stressed out is very uncomfortable, and it's only natural to look for ways to feel better. It's quick and easy to find momentary relief by eating palatable food, smoking cigarettes, or drinking excessively.

Another strategy people often use to deal with stress is avoidance and numbing out by surfing the internet or watching television for hours every day. All of these habits are risk factors for one chronic disease or another and most people know this, but they grow reliant on these quick fixes and distractions for stress relief and have a hard time giving them up.

A good way to start understanding your own ways of coping is through self-monitoring of your "bad" habits. If you smoke cigarettes, drink a bit too much alcohol, eat junk food, or spend too much time on the couch, it would be helpful to examine what thoughts, feelings, and/or events lead to these behaviors. Do the two-day coping assessment: every time you engage in one of your "vices," take a moment to note that you're doing it and jot down how you're feeling at the time. See if you can identify consistent triggers for these activities and over time, you'll be able to come up with alternatives.

In this book, you'll learn some specific ways to improve your skill at both types of coping—problem management and emotional regulation. They're both important because they help you alleviate your stress physiology in the moment, and they will help you start to put life's challenges into a more manageable perspective so you aren't so easily pushed into unhealthy emotional states. Belly fat and stress go together closely. The better you are at cutting down your stress responses, the more quickly and easily you'll lose your belly.

How Stress Changes Physiology

The second pathway from stress to disease is through the direct effects of the hormones the body makes as part of the stress response. Your body's physical response to psychological stress is perfectly designed to deal with a potentially catastrophic emergency that is short-lived and with longer lasting difficulty like the seasonal famine faced by hunter-gatherers.

Unfortunately, the stressors we face in the modern world can last for years and years in the case of a bad job, financial hardship, or a dysfunctional marriage. These types of hassles and problems keep your body's stress system simmering away, pushing many of your cells and organs much harder than they can tolerate without harm.

RED FLAG

Chronic stress creeps up on us as years of daily disappointments, worries, fears, and regrets pile up. What many think of as normal aging, such as aches and pains, headaches, fatigue, insomnia, and poor digestion are often actually the cumulative effects of stress and poor coping. If you have some or most of these common complaints, you're probably in need of some good coping skills.

How does modern-day stress differ from the primitive types of stress we're designed to endure?

- Because modern-day stressors are primarily psychological, social, and emotional, they are not paired with the extreme physical exertion required to metabolize all the sugar and fat mobilized by the stress response.

- Modern-day stressors tend to be either prolonged (e.g., unemployment, unhappy marriages, caring for a sick spouse or child) or repetitive (daily hassles at work, a long commute) and therefore trigger frequent and/or continuous activation of the stress response.

- Modern-day chronic stress occurs in an environment that is teeming with readily available, inexpensive, and highly palatable food.

- Modern-day stress occurs in environments and situations where physical activity is easily avoided and readily replaced with passive, avoidant, and sedentary activities.

What Is Stress, Anyway?

Let's examine the basic biology of stress and how it leads to fat in the belly. People who are chronically stressed have elevated levels of two basic hormones in their body—*adrenaline* (also called epinephrine) and *cortisol*. They also have constant low-level activation of the part of the nervous system that's in charge of fear-based behavior—fight or flight—called the sympathetic nervous system. Cortisol comes from the adrenal glands. Adrenaline comes from the adrenal glands and the fibers of the sympathetic nervous system. Both have profound affects in the body.

DEFINITION

Cortisol is a steroid hormone produced and secreted by the adrenal glands, which are located on top of your kidneys. Cortisol is released into the blood-stream and circulates all over the body, causing long-lasting changes in many cells and organs. **Adrenaline** is a short-acting hormone released by the adrenal glands and nervous system in an acute stress response. It produces many of the changes familiar to many as an "adrenaline rush," such as elevations in heart rate and blood pressure, cold hands and feet, and sweating.

These two major chemicals of stress have different effects, but they work in tandem to keep you on high alert, even when you're not in a dangerous situation. All you have to do is think about something that you're worried about, and the whole stress system gets turned on. This is how people differ from all other animals—we can think ourselves into a full-blown stress response—one that was designed to be used only in case of true life-threatening emergencies, and only on rare occasions.

Adrenaline is a quick acting molecule that creates the "adrenaline rush" of a sudden scare or startle or emergency. It has powerful, immediate effects on every system of our bodies—but the most dangerous effects are elevation of heart rate and blood pressure. During the course of our lifetimes, about 90 percent of us will develop high blood pressure. Stress is frequently either the cause or a contributing factor to this.

Cortisol is a long-lasting steroid hormone that has profound effects on how your body acquires, processes, stores, and expends energy. Energy comes from food—which means that cortisol is a major player in regulating your appetite and energy levels—and how much fat you're storing, and where that fat is being stored.

Stress and Cortisol

It's easy to understand cortisol's role in energy, metabolism, and fat deposition when you consider that the stress response we are wired with is the same one that helped untold generations of hunter-gatherer humans survive the hazards of prehistoric life.

Hunter-gatherers faced three primary threats to their well-being and survival. First, they had to be able to defend themselves and their families from any kind of physical assault, be it from other humans, predators, the animals they were hunting, or a harsh environment. That's the fight function. Second, they had to expend huge bursts of energy at any given time—to chase down an animal for food, and to escape fights and assaults they had no chance of surviving. This is the flight function. Finally, hunter-gatherers had to go out and walk or run, sometimes great distances, for days and possibly weeks at a time searching for food. This is the famine function.

WHAT'S NEW

Hunter-gatherers were humans living during the Paleolithic Era (45,000 to 12,000 years ago), before the invention of agriculture. Recent research is debunking the common image of the grunting caveman—hunter-gatherers used tools and created art, developed sophisticated and protective social networks, and made good use of fire. Genetic science has shown that our DNA hasn't changed much if at all since those days, so we're all "cavemen" to some extent, living in an alien, modern world.

All three of these functions require the same set of changes in the body. The primary need for fight, flee, or famine is to provide the muscles with as much energy as possible. Muscles use fat and sugar, primarily, to generate movement. These fuels come from food, of course. A routine everyday intake of food is perfectly adequate to provide energy for routine days. However, when a severe threat arises, whether it's sudden or gradual, the body needs to mobilize a huge increase in these fuels over its everyday needs. Cortisol is the supervisor of this mobilization.

Cortisol's mission is to increase blood levels of fat and sugar as quickly as possible for fight, flight, or famine. To do this, cortisol's overall effect is to shut down or suppress all bodily functions involved in growth, development, and long-term well-being to allocate all available energy and raw materials to bodily processes involved in emergency responses. In addition, cortisol acts on the liver and fat stores to release as much fuel as possible for use by the skeletal muscles and brain.

To these ends, cortisol has these direct effects on the cells and organs of the body:

- Interacts with appetite centers in the brain to initially suppress but chronically stimulate appetite for food

- Stimulates production and release of glucose by the liver, leading to a large increase in blood sugar

- Suppresses the ability of insulin receptors to respond to the high levels of insulin that are released by the pancreas in response to the blood sugar surge

- Stimulates immune functions related to inflammation and wound healing

- Suppresses immune functions related to sophisticated responses to viral infections

- Suppresses release of human growth hormone (HGH) from the pituitary gland, clearing the way for breakdown of muscle and even bone to provide fuel for fight, flight, or famine

- Suppresses release of sex steroids, thus inhibiting sexual behavior and, in women, ovulation and pregnancy

- Triggers breakdown of fat in subcutaneous stores (hips, thighs, etc.), thus increasing the amount of fat circulating in the blood

In the short term, all of these actions of cortisol are adaptive and beneficial. They make it possible for those superhuman acts that can save lives in an emergency. They are all perfectly appropriate for dealing with the three basic stressors faced by hunter-gatherers, but they are very damaging and inappropriate for the types of stressors faced by modern men and women.

From Stress to Disease

So let's take a snapshot at the average stressed-out American woman in her 40s. For one reason or another, she thinks she's unable to effectively cope with all the demands of her life, which she's come to perceive as unrelenting and uncontrollable. These thoughts make her feel afraid that she will eventually fail at one or more of her roles in life, and angry that so much has been put on her shoulders. She's also aware that her problems will never magically disappear, and she will always be coping with them, or another set of problems. This idea makes her feel hopeless and anxious.

Emotions and Stress

Our stressed friend now has a whole package of negative emotions that were generated by her thoughts about the stressful events and circumstances of her life. Negative emotions trigger the stress response. This makes sense when you consider what sorts of things most likely caused anxiety, sadness, or fear in a person living in prehistoric times. Not taxes! Much like the stress response, negative emotions appeared and persisted in the human experience as a matter of survival. One can imagine a prolonged famine would evoke anxiety, and the sight of an approaching aggressor would generate fear or anger or both.

Fear, anger, and anxious sadness are all potential triggers of full-blown stress responses. So our friend now has elevated cortisol levels and chronic activation of her sympathetic nervous system along with her unhappiness.

Fight or Flight

Chronic sympathetic activation puts a person into a mild form of fight or flight. Heart rate, blood pressure, and respiratory rate are increased and stay that way, putting immense mechanical and metabolic pressure on the cardiovascular system. Blood flow is shunted preferentially to the skeletal muscles and the head, inducing chronic muscle tension and frequent stress and migraine headaches.

Shunting blood to the head and muscles requires persistent shunting of blood away from the digestive organs. This can cause all kinds of gastrointestinal symptoms, from heartburn to bloating and gassiness, loose stools or constipation.

Considering all these negative physical effects it's not surprising that the Centers for Disease Control (CDC), a government agency devoted to protecting, promoting, and monitoring public health and safety, estimates that about 75 percent of outpatient doctor visits are for conditions either caused by or exacerbated by stress. In our modern age, job stress is particularly common, and has been directly connected to an elevated risk for cardiovascular disease, musculoskeletal disorders, psychological problems, and injuries at work.

RED FLAG

If your job is driving you crazy, it's not something to take lightly. The CDC recommends stress management training for individuals and organization-level changes such as workload reduction, making schedules more regular and controllable, and promoting good relationships as ways to address workplace stress and its dangers.

That sounds pretty uncomfortable, doesn't it? Also pretty common in the average American adult. But that's only half the story.

The adrenal gland is busy putting out cortisol at higher than normal amounts in response to an adult's persistent negative emotions and fearful thoughts. The hypothalamus cannot discern the difference between his fearful thoughts about an imminent attack on his person and fearful thoughts about not being able to make next month's car payment. It is wired, along with other parts of the brain, to simply detect fear.

As long as the adult continues feeling angry, anxious, and fearful, his lower brain and stress system will continue to respond to those thoughts and feelings with survival-level functions. Looking again at the list of effects cortisol has on the body, you can make some pretty accurate assumptions about his behaviors and risk factors for disease.

Stress, Food, and Getting Fat

When people are feeling stressed and overwhelmed, they often turn toward food for comfort. This leads to many people overeating (especially comfort foods) and feeling disinclined to exercise or extend themselves socially. These behaviors all serve the purpose of maintaining or increasing bodily energy reserves. The hypothalamus, while not part of the brain that makes choices and decisions, can send messages that steer our thought processes toward food and away from exercising.

Remember palatability? This is something the famine-stressed hunter-gatherer seeks and devours, because she's energy deficient, perhaps even starving. Our modern day hunter-gatherer is driven, just like her ancient ancestor, to seek and consume highly palatable food. Remember, the stress response exists as much to induce persistent food-seeking behavior in a famine as it does to ready the body for fight or flight.

GOOD MOVE

If you tend to eat candy, pastries, or salty snacks when you're stressed, you aren't alone. It's estimated that about ⅓ of women and 20 percent of men do this. Start cutting back on this habit right now by replacing your usual stress snack with a small handful—about 15 to 20—of raw almonds and/or a cup of fresh berries. These tidbits are palatable but also healthy, and can give you that little bit of mouth comfort without drastically plumping your belly.

So now our friend is eating more than usual and choosing more palatable food, which is higher in calories, fat, and sweeteners than the food she normally eats. She is able to consume many excess calories every day because there's palatable food everywhere she goes, including the gas station!

All day now, she is putting unneeded excess fuel into her body, which is now programmed to hold on to every calorie in the form of fat. Her body is also programmed by cortisol to store that fat in a place where it's easily released if and when the imminent threat to survival materializes—inside her abdomen.

Cortisol Raises Blood Sugar and Fat

Meanwhile, cortisol is busy keeping her blood sugar high in two basic ways. It's stimulating the liver to mobilize and release large amounts of sugar into her bloodstream. It's also interacting with insulin receptors, primarily in the liver and skeletal muscles, to make them resistant to the effects of the insulin in the blood. Blood insulin levels are high, because the liver is maintaining elevated blood sugar.

When both insulin and cortisol are elevated, they exert even more pressure on the body to shift fat stores from subcutaneous locations such as the hips and buttocks to the belly. That way, when the looming physical catastrophe that the body is expecting finally occurs, blood lipid levels will be easily and dramatically elevated to fuel fight or flight.

So our friend's body shape is gradually but surely transforming from a healthy pear to an unhealthy apple. Her belly fat is growing a little more each day.

Chronically elevated blood sugar and insulin, paired with long-term *insulin receptor resistance* leads to *impaired glucose tolerance*. This means that any additional load of sugar that appears from the diet will not be readily cleared from the blood, making the whole problem even worse. Over time, impaired glucose tolerance leads to full-blown Type 2 diabetes if nothing is done to remedy the situation.

DEFINITION

Impaired glucose tolerance (IGT) is a condition that develops over time because of **insulin receptor resistance,** which refers to changes in the receptors for insulin in your skeletal muscle and fat leading them to become scarcer and less prone to allow insulin to bind to them. If insulin can't bind to its receptors, the cells can't take up blood sugar, so blood sugar stays high, making a person unable to "tolerate" a large intake of carbohydrates. Without significant changes in lifestyle, IGT is very likely to develop into Type 2 diabetes.

The continued breakdown of subcutaneous fat keeps blood levels of triglycerides elevated, making the blood thicker and more prone to clotting. Elevated triglycerides also direct the liver to produce more artery-damaging LDL.

Stress and Inflammation

Our poor friend has by now built up a big mass of intra-abdominal fat rich with macrophages that are pumping out chemicals that are stimulating other macrophages all over her body, including ones that are located in the arteries of her heart. These macrophages are itching for a fight—and fighting for them involves grabbing and gobbling up any cell or molecule that it thinks is a little bit out of the ordinary.

LDL levels are abnormally high because of the continued release of triglycerides from the peripheral fat stores, so more LDL is entering the walls of the coronary artery than usual. Arterial blood, rich in oxygen, is coursing through these arteries. Now here's one more piece of the puzzle.

Oxidative Stress and Diet

While oxygen is essential to life, when it participates in the metabolic processes of the cells of our bodies, it is transformed into a potentially harmful version of itself called a reactive oxygen species (ROS). These particles have an electric charge, which makes it easy for them to stick to various structures inside the cells, including DNA. When ROS particles aren't eliminated promptly and start binding to DNA and cell membranes, this is called oxidative damage.

In a healthy, well-nourished body, there are enzymes standing by all the time, ready to make quick work of the ROS particles, converting them back into good old oxygen before they can get unruly and start damaging the cells. These enzymes require the presence of other small molecules in order to work. Have you guessed what these particles are?

If you guessed antioxidants, you're right. Antioxidants are molecules that help deactivate ROS particles by becoming oxidized themselves, thus preventing damage to other cells. Of the many antioxidants found in food, some of the most potent are vitamin C, vitamin A, selenium, and zinc. Because our bodies are incapable of producing antioxidants, they must come from our diet. Furthermore, most of them work best as a team, meaning together they are stronger than each one individually.

WHAT'S NEW

Several studies looking at the ability of supplements to prevent disease have had poor results—but this is because most studies focused on giving one antioxidant at a time. As you learn more about these vital nutrients, you see that they work synergistically. To reap their benefits, you need to get them from whole food supplements or, best of all, the foods themselves.

Not surprisingly, antioxidants come from the plants that used to comprise more than ¾ of the human diet—for more than 95 percent of the time humans have been on the planet. As long as your diet contains plenty of fruits and vegetables, nuts, whole grains, and lean, clean protein, you'll have plenty of antioxidant nutrients to prevent any buildup of ROS in your cells.

Stress, Fat, and Your Heart

Okay—getting back to our unfortunate friend—remember that stress and negative emotions have caused her to change her diet from one that was reasonably healthy to one high in junk food and low in the very foods she needs to protect herself from the effects of stress.

Now let's put all the players together in the wall of one of this woman's coronary arteries. You have a crowd of LDL particles pushing and shoving their way into the artery wall in numbers much higher than normal. You have a gang of grumpy macrophages, over-stimulated by the cytokines being sent their way by their brothers living in her belly fat.

The cells of the artery wall aren't all too happy, either. You see, glucose, like oxygen and LDL, is necessary for cells to survive. But too much glucose is an irritant to cells, and stresses them. When the cells lining an artery are stressed, they don't function as well as they normally do. You'll remember that our friend has chronically elevated blood glucose because her high levels of cortisol have disabled her insulin receptors, so the sugar has no way of moving from her bloodstream into her cells to feed them.

The irritated, stressed cells lining the coronary artery get along as well as they can, but their metabolic processes are continually generating ROS species. Unfortunately, these cells are further at a disadvantage because our friend's diet is almost devoid of antioxidants at this point, so ROS particles are building up in the artery wall. It doesn't take long for the sluggish, overcrowded LDLs to bump into the highly reactive ROS particles, which promptly bind to them in a process called oxidation.

When perfectly innocent molecules in the body undergo oxidation, they are no longer functional and they're potentially harmful. For example, ROS binding to the DNA of a cell can so derange its function that it converts the normal body cell into a cancer cell. The potential harm that oxidized molecules can wreak on the body make them prime targets for elimination by macrophages. After all, it's their job to hunt down all abnormal, injured, or dysfunctional cells and particles in addition to killing bacteria.

The macrophages in the artery wall dutifully start gobbling up the oxidized LDLs. Unfortunately, they can't digest or break these particles down. So the whole mess—a blob of rancid LDLs packed inside activated, overstuffed macrophages gets lodged in the artery wall forming what we call atherosclerotic plaque—the basic defect in coronary artery disease. This process continues for years, even decades, until the plaque cracks open, causing the blood in the artery to clot. The clot moves downstream and gets stuck in a narrower section of artery. This stops all blood flow to the heart muscle beyond the plaque. The heart muscle will die unless our friend gets immediate medical care.

As you've seen, poorly managed stress can lead to a whole series of potentially dangerous changes in your thoughts, emotions, and physiology—all of which can set you up for heart disease and other medical problems. The program in this book provides you not only with good advice about what to eat and how to exercise, but also with powerful, effective new ways to minimize the damage stress can do.

The Least You Need to Know

- Stress arises when you perceive life's challenges as threats to your well-being that you aren't fully able to cope with.
- Stress leads to unhealthy, feel-good behaviors such as eating comfort food and retreating to your couch.
- Stress physiology, known as fight or flight, is caused by an increase in cortisol and activation of your sympathetic nervous system.
- Chronically activated stress responses increase your risk of disease by elevating blood lipids and sugar, aggravating your immune system's inflammatory cells, and accelerating oxidative damage to your cells.

Your New Food Lifestyle

Changing the way you eat and your attitude about food is an important step in losing belly fat and keeping it off. It's not about going on or off a diet. It's about learning to love whole, natural, healthy foods that make you feel and look better. In this part we'll discuss all the foods you should be eating—good carbs, good fats, and plenty of protein—and all the foods and drinks you should avoid—saturated fat, sugary beverages, and salty foods. We'll also spend some time talking about the Mediterranean diet, a model eating plan that can improve health, help you live longer, and trim down your middle.

A Program for Life

In This Chapter

- Discovering the problem with diets
- Developing a good attitude
- Avoiding belly bloaters
- Discovering the wonderful world of healthy food

For hunter-gatherers, belly fat was vital for surviving lean times when food was scarce. This pooch (belly fat) produced a cascade of physiological changes that were necessary for us to thrive in a Paleolithic environment. In modern times, however, our genetic tendency to eat as much as we can of highly palatable food and then store it as belly fat is not an advantage. Combined with low levels of physical activity and high levels of stress, these excess calories cause us bulging bellies that are not only unhealthy but can lead to a variety of chronic illnesses such as heart disease, Type 2 diabetes, and high blood pressure.

The good news is it doesn't have to be that way. You can lose this belly fat—and keep it off—without feeling deprived, starved, or stressed. All it takes is the right attitude and a willingness to make a change—this doesn't mean dieting. In this chapter you learn how to decrease your belly fat without "dieting," how to choose foods that will keep your waist slim and trim, and avoid foods that don't. More importantly, you'll be able to take this new knowledge and adapt it to your own lifestyle so the changes you make are changes you can live with and are realistic.

All Weight-Loss Diets Are Temporary

Many people think the only way to lose weight is to go on a weight-loss "diet," but these types of diets just don't work. If they did, we would be a nation of svelte, thin, or normal weight individuals—but unfortunately that's not the case. In fact, more of us are overweight and obese than normal weight, and our penchant for going on "weight-loss diets" may in part be responsible.

So why doesn't the weight we lose on weight-loss diets last? Some of this has to do with our own attitude and commitment, and some has to do with the nature of the weight-loss diet itself. For most people, "dieting" and weight loss is a temporary goal, meaning people often see diets as something they will go on and then off as soon as they reach their desired weight. The problem is that after they're "off" the diet, most people go right back to eating exactly as they did before—wolfing down high calorie, highly processed fatty foods—and that leads to gaining back the weight lost.

Secondly, few weight-loss diets are actually designed to produce a lifestyle change. Rather they are a prescribed plan, usually rigid in nature, that doesn't take into account personal likes and dislikes or individual eating habits and often promotes repetitive food patterns. Thus, at best, most offer only short-term solutions to a long-term problem.

Finally, many weight-loss diets offer quick-fixes and make unrealistic promises. These are fad diets. You can spot a *fad diet* by looking for one or more of the following features:

- Overemphasis of a specific food or dish, like the grapefruit diet, the cabbage soup diet, or the juice diet

- An imbalance of nutrients—low fat, low carb, high protein, etc.

- Little if any physical activity

- Liquid supplements or meal replacements

 DEFINITION

Fad diets are popular weight-loss plans that promise quick weight loss by severely limiting certain foods and overemphasizing others.

The Statistics of Dieting

Because most weight-loss diets are more concerned with cutting calories than teaching people a better and healthier way to eat, most people who follow a weight-loss diet are not successful.

So although dieters will initially lose 5 to 10 percent of their body weight (mostly belly fat) on any number of meal plans, the weight typically comes right back, usually within a few years' time. This leads to more dieting and an unhealthy cycle of losing and gaining weight, known as yo-yo dieting, which can cause even greater weight gain than before. To break this cycle, you need to focus not on cutting calories but on developing your own healthy meal pattern, which includes choosing a variety of healthy foods to eat, eating at regular times, and getting enough daily physical activity. We'll cover more about the specifics of what's in a healthy meal plan in Chapters 5 and 6.

WHAT'S NEW

Each year approximately 50 million Americans go on a diet—yet only 5 percent keep the weight they lose off for more than five years.

Too Much Restriction Can Lead to Weight Gain

Some fad diets are called crash diets because they promote severe calorie restriction. These diets are particularly unhealthy because they strive to do the exact opposite of what our bodies have evolved to do over thousands of years when calories were scarce—conserve energy. Consequently it's no surprise that they are nearly impossible to follow, for even short periods of time, have a low success rate, and ultimately end up adding on more pounds than they took off.

During times of famine (or when on a crash diet), your body is hard-wired to switch into low gear. This low gear is designed to use as little energy as possible so you can survive until the next time abundant food is available, which during Paleolithic times could last for days or even weeks. Metabolism slows, heart rate slows, and the body struggles to sparingly use the energy it stored as fat, meaning fat breakdown decreases. Appetite is suppressed as well, so your desire for food drops and lethargy sets in, further decreasing energy output.

At the same time, to compensate for fewer calories, protein breakdown increases and normal cell reproduction decreases, lowering your resistance to disease and reducing practically all non-vital functions (such as growing hair or nails).

When food finally does become available (i.e., you go off the crash diet), your body doesn't immediately bounce back. Appetite increases quickly and you often crave high calorie, palatable food as your body seeks to replace the calories it lost. But, metabolism stays low sometimes for months or even years afterward. Protein losses and fat stores are restored and may even be ramped up in case such an "emergency" happens again. Low energy output (metabolism) combined with high energy input (an insatiable appetite) results in weight gain, often above and beyond what you originally started with. Studies show that for both men and women, those who participate in formal weight-loss programs have a greater chance of putting on more weight than those who didn't try to lose weight.

GOOD MOVE

To avoid yo-yo dieting, nix fad diets and instead focus on small changes that make a difference, like eating more whole natural foods, skipping processed foods, and switching from high-fat, high-calorie foods to lower ones—such as choosing broiled chicken instead of fried. Set realistic weight-loss goals and plan on cutting about 250 to 500 calories a day while upping your physical activity. This should give you a 1- to 2-pound weight loss a week.

Lose the All-or-Nothing Attitude

When it comes to losing belly fat, having an all-or-nothing attitude is a sure way to set yourself up for failure. With no room for an occasional mistake or sweet treat, all-or-nothing dieters often end up going overboard after a single slip-up and bingeing on rich, sugary, or fatty foods, bringing their dieting days quickly to an end. Worse yet is the fact that this also can lead to an emotional rollercoaster ride, with dieters constantly beating themselves up for failing.

Rather than fall into this negative cycle, think of your weight-loss plan as a journey or process of small steps. Each step is a success that should be celebrated and enjoyed. Occasional setbacks are simply that, an occasional setback. Allow yourself to splurge a meal or two or even a few day's worth of food, but then get back on track. Life happens. Concentrate on the positives rather than the negatives—how much weight or inches you've already lost—and move forward from there. Don't lose sight of your goal. Remember you're making healthy lifestyle changes to last a lifetime. It's the small steps that turn into long-term changes that matter.

Think Abundance, Not Deprivation

Many people think going on a weight-loss diet means skimpy portions and bland food. Nothing could be further from the truth. Your plate will be filled with colorful vegetables, fruits, beans and legumes, and whole grains complemented with a wide array of fresh flavorful herbs and spices. Because these foods are naturally low in calories and high in fiber, you can easily eat hefty portion sizes without gaining weight and are more likely to end up losing weight and inches. Check out the recipes in Chapters 16 through 21 for some good meal ideas.

But even though the majority of your meals will be fresh, healthy, wholesome food, this doesn't mean you can't enjoy your favorite high-calorie food, sweet treat, or snack once in a while. Let's face it—everyone has food cravings and the food you crave isn't likely to be the best kind for you. Giving in to these cravings *once in a while* is key to having a successful, healthy meal plan. In fact, studies show dieters who occasionally give in to food cravings are more likely to stay on their diet and lose weight than those who don't give in.

RED FLAG

Don't give in to every food craving that comes along, rather take a walk (exercise is great for relieving cravings), call someone, or simply wait it out—sometimes cravings lessen with time. If you do give in, make sure it is worth your while and choose only the best, high-quality product you can find.

Staying the Course

Humans are creatures of habit, so whenever you provoke a change in eating habits or anything else there's sure to be a fair share of ups and downs. Eating patterns are particularly difficult to alter because the foods we choose are ingrained in our genetic make-up as well as determined by a multitude of emotional and behavioral factors. Nevertheless, you can make a change and learn to appreciate, enjoy, and value wholesome, healthy, unprocessed foods similar to what our ancestors thrived on as long as you are committed. Remember, too, you don't have to overhaul your diet overnight.

Small steps are important—like switching from whole milk to skim or adding more beans to your diet—and can add up to big changes over time.

The key is to keep your eye on the long-term goal—staying fit and healthy and feeling good about yourself and your body.

Eliminate Belly Bloaters

A bloated belly is a common condition for many people and it doesn't feel good. You're uncomfortable, distended, and often gassy. Stress, lack of sleep, and dehydration can trigger belly bloat but so can certain foods. Luckily the same foods you would avoid to keep your belly bloat at bay are foods you'd want to watch out for on any healthy diet. So not only are you doing your belly good, you're also helping your heart and reducing your risk of high blood pressure, diabetes, and obesity.

Simple Sugars and Refined Carbs

Carbohydrates are classified based on how many monosaccharide units they contain. A monosaccharide—glucose, for example—is the simplest of sugars, composed of a single carbohydrate molecule. A disaccharide has two molecules bound together. Polysaccharides such as fiber and starch are made of hundreds or even thousands of sugar molecules strung together.

Natural sugars tend to be disaccharides. Sucrose, or table sugar, is a disaccharide made of glucose and fructose. It's quickly broken down by the digestive system into its two constituent monosaccharides. The glucose passes directly from the intestine into the bloodstream while the fructose travels to the liver for processing there.

In the hunter-gatherer diet, there was very little sucrose or *simple sugar* in the diet. In our modern world, we eat a lot of it—more than 22 teaspoons of added sugars, or 350 calories worth, (added sugars include sucrose, white table sugar, dextrose, high fructose corn syrup, brown sugar, honey, molasses, turbinado, and more) a day. Most of these sugars are *refined*, meaning purified during processing. In Paleolithic times, sugar was available primarily from fruits, and sugar in fruit comes with a good dose of fiber, which slows down its absorption. Today, the majority of our added sugars comes to us in beverages—soft drinks, energy drinks, and sports drinks. These sugars are quickly absorbed, causing rapid, drastic increases in blood sugar and insulin levels (we'll talk more about insulin in Chapter 6).

DEFINITION

Simple sugars are readily absorbed by the body. The main ones are sucrose (table sugar), fructose, and lactose. **Refined sugars** are stripped of all nutrients during processing. White table sugar, cane sugar, and high fructose corn syrup are refined sugars.

There is currently a great deal of controversy and research focused on the relative dangers of sugar and high fructose corn syrup (HFCS), as we saw in Chapter 1. The data are mixed, but one thing remains clear. Because inexpensive HFCS not only functions as a sweetener, but also as a palatability enhancer and food stabilizer, it's added to just about every food manufactured in the United States today.

Because sweeteners are in almost all processed foods, which make up the bulk of most people's diets, we have seen a huge shift in our food preferences toward sweetness. In fact the more sugar you eat, the more sweetness you crave. The good news is you can learn to control this tendency toward sweetness by cutting the sugar out. Eventually you won't even miss the sugar, but this won't happen overnight, it may take weeks or even months for your taste buds to adjust.

GOOD MOVE

People who have a sweet tooth may find it very hard to give up their sweets. At first, food tends to seem bland, sour, bitter, or just unpleasant. But, this doesn't last long. Keep to the plan and you'll soon learn to love the natural, wholesome flavor of unadulterated food while you watch your belly get steadily smaller.

Sugars contribute to weight problems and risk factors for diabetes. They add empty calories to food, stimulate overly aggressive insulin responses to eating, and in the case of HFCS, induce accumulation of fat in the liver, leading to harmful changes in the liver's management of blood sugar and blood lipids. All of these effects contribute to the buildup of belly fat.

As with purified simple sugar, refined sugars and *refined carbohydrates* such as white flour, white bread, and white pasta are concentrated sources of calories with little nutritional value. And, like simple sugar, refined carbohydrates elevate blood sugar levels and increase insulin response.

DEFINITION

Refined carbohydrates are foods that have been modified to enhance shelf life or make them easier to eat or digest. Refined carbohydrates are generally in the form of white flour, where the bran and the germ of the whole grain are removed, and only the endosperm remains intact.

Eating high levels of both simple sugars and refined carbohydrates are associated with larger waistlines and bloated bellies. What's the bottom line? Sans the sugars and carbs by getting rid of processed foods and drinks with added sugar. Instead look for complex carbohydrates like whole grains and acquire a taste for natural sugars in fruit. If you do want to add some sweetness to your cereal or vegetables, don't use more than a teaspoon or two of sugar or honey per person per day. One teaspoon of sugar contains 16 calories and one teaspoon of honey contains 21 calories—this can add up quickly throughout the course of a day.

Fats to Avoid

Trans fats are a man-made fat that has been linked to a whole host of health problems, so it's not surprising that this is one fat you should definitely avoid for controlling belly fat.

As with simple sugars and refined carbohydrates, trans fats are found only in processed foods, so if you stay away from them you're sure to stay away from trans fats. On ingredient labels, trans fats are listed as "partially hydrogenated" or as "hydrogenated" oils. Ultimately, it doesn't matter whether it's corn, soybean, or some other oil that's been hydrogenated. What's important is to know that hydrogenation creates trans fats, and they're not good for you. And don't just look on the nutrition label. Manufacturers are allowed to say a food has no trans fats even if the product contains them, as long as each serving contains less than .5 grams. So if you eat more than one serving or several products with trans fats in them, you're probably getting more than you know.

Certain saturated fats found in meat and high-fat dairy products can also be dangerous to your health and your waistline. This is why the flat belly diet recommends keeping red meat and dairy products to a minimum (more about this in Chapter 5). If you do want to include these foods in your diet, go for grass-fed rather than corn-fed animals. Not only are the animals treated better, but the grass-fed animals produce a better, healthier fatty acid profile. And be sure to choose low-fat dairy products such as skim milk or nonfat yogurt.

Too Much Salt

When it comes to belly bloat, salt is one of the main culprits. Salt is composed of 40 percent sodium and 60 percent chloride. In the body sodium attracts water, so the more sodium you have in your body the more water you have. This leads to not only extra water weight but a puffy or swollen appearance in your belly and elsewhere, and a sluggish feeling throughout the day. If you think part of your belly bloat is due to the amount of salt you're eating, take note of the foods you're eating right before you feel swollen and think twice about having those foods.

Remember, too, that not all foods that are high in salt taste salty. Much of the salt in processed foods such as ketchup and soups is "hidden." Over the years, people who follow a typical American diet have grown so accustomed to high levels of salt, that sometimes they can barely notice if a food tastes salty or not. Although sodium levels vary depending on the size and shape of the salt crystal, on average one-quarter teaspoon of fine grained table salt contains about 575 milligrams of sodium. You want to aim to keep sodium consumption below 2,300 milligrams a day.

GOOD MOVE

If you want to avoid salt, pass over processed foods (anything in a box, bag, or can) and aim for all fresh, whole natural foods. Seventy-five percent of our salt intake comes from processed foods.

If you want to control your salt intake, skip the frozen dinner or boxed macaroni and cheese and use the salt shaker on whole foods you've prepared instead. People who salt their food at the table typically use much less salt than the salt used in food processing. Furthermore, because the salt is on top of the food and touches the tongue first, the salt taste is more pronounced, making for a more satisfying food experience.

Focus on Healthy Food

Many people rely on processed foods for most of their meals. To reduce belly fat you want to instead focus on whole, natural, unprocessed foods—fresh produce; fresh meat, fish, and poultry; and whole grains, legumes, and beans. To do this you need to first do three things.

1. **Stock up on healthy food.** Go to the grocery store and fill your cart with fresh fruits, vegetables, and meat. Be sure and plan your menu before going to the store, as fresh foods are more perishable than processed or manufactured foods.

2. **Get rid of all your junk food.** This includes nearly all of your mixes; packaged side dishes; prepared frozen snacks, starches, and desserts; and sugary cereals. These foods are loaded with fat, sugar, and salt as well as a host of artificial ingredients. In addition to making room for all the healthy foods you will buy, getting rid of this junk food will also remove temptation and create a safe food environment.

3. **Learn to cook.** There's no way around it, when you start eating a healthier diet and get rid of processed convenience foods, you have to get to know your way around the kitchen. Buy some good knives, a cutting board, and good quality pots and pans. Then just begin chopping away. If you're really unsure of yourself or need a boost of confidence, take a cooking course or two, or ask a friend who's good in the kitchen to give you some pointers.

The World of Good Healthy Food

Healthy food is all around you, it's just a matter of opening your eyes to find it. In the grocery store, focus on healthy, all-natural food. Make the first stop in your grocery store in the fresh produce department. Instead of protein, think about centering at least one of your next few meals around a vegetable.

Experiment with new vegetables or fruits you haven't seen before. Many stores now have different ethnic sections in their produce department, so consider exploring that as well.

If you don't find what you need in the produce section, check out frozen vegetables. They're just as nutritious as fresh in most cases. Just be sure to read the label to be sure there is no extra salt or sugar added.

Next, move on to the fresh meat, poultry, and fish aisles. Beware of meats that have been pre-seasoned, sauced, or pre-cooked. These foods are highly processed, expensive, and loaded with sugar, salt, and unwanted preservatives and additives.

RED FLAG

Steer clear of fresh meat or poultry that says it's "enhanced with 15 percent solution" or "contains up to 15 percent natural chicken broth." This means the chicken or meat was injected with a salt-sugar or salt solution, which can more than double the sodium naturally found in fresh meat.

In the seafood department, choose wild-caught over farm-raised, and buy both shell-fish and finfish. But beware of big fish like shark, swordfish, tilefish, and some types of tuna, which may have higher mercury levels or other contaminants. For the best environmentally conscious choices, look at Monterey Bay Aquarium's Seafood Watch Guide (see Appendix B), which is specific to each region of the country.

Stock up on nuts (roasted unsalted); whole grains like brown rice, quinoa, barley, and whole-grain couscous; legumes and beans (dried are best); and good monounsaturated fats like avocado, olive oil, and peanut oil.

How to Select the Best

Because wholesome, healthy food tends to be more perishable and fragile than convenience food, it pays to buy the best quality possible. Check produce carefully for bumps and bruises and don't assume if something doesn't look attractive it isn't good. This is particularly the case at local farmers' markets where produce often doesn't look as pretty as conventional grocery store products, particularly when it comes to heirloom fruits and vegetables. Here are some other tips:

- **Buy in season.** Seasonal produce is fresher and cheaper than produce bought out of season. It also tastes better.

- **Use it right away.** Unlike processed or packaged foods that can sit on the shelves for months, fresh foods go bad quickly.

- **Handle fresh foods with care.** Refrigerate produce, proteins, and dairy immediately and always wrap properly. Dry goods need to be stored in a cool dry place.

- **Search out local markets.** Local farmers' markets, farm stores, and food co-ops offer fresh wholesome food straight from the farm. This is also a great place to find grass-fed meats and high-quality eggs. Not only will you find high-quality fresh food at these markets but you can also find more variety and products that you can't get elsewhere. Sometimes you can even get better prices, too, as there is no middleman.

- **Read food labels.** Food labels tell you both the nutrition information and the ingredients in a specific product. They're vital for determining if the food or ingredient fits into your healthy meal plan. As a general rule, try to avoid labels with ingredients you don't recognize.

The Least You Need to Know

- The best way to lose belly fat is to make small changes to your eating habits, be flexible, and adapt these changes to your lifestyle over time.

- Fad diets focusing on calorie restriction and deprivation don't work. Instead focus on long-term goals and don't beat yourself up about occasional slip-ups.

- To lose belly fat and reduce bloating, cut out foods with refined white flour, added sugars, trans fats, and lots of salt.

- A healthful diet that slims your belly includes wholesome, natural foods like fresh produce; whole grains, legumes, beans, and nuts; lean meat, including chicken, pork, turkey, and roast beef; and fish. All these foods are readily available at the grocery store and local markets.

Eat to Burn Fat

In This Chapter

* The magic of the Mediterranean diet
* A rundown of healthy fats: MUFAs and more
* Protein to keep you satisfied
* High protein foods to keep your belly in check

When it comes to modern diets, the Mediterranean eating pattern just may be the best kind of diet for shedding belly fat and staying healthy. Study after study shows people who eat this way can combat heart disease, stroke, certain cancers, diabetes, and metabolic syndrome better than people who don't.

The main difference between the Med diet and the typical American diet is that the Med diet limits potentially harmful saturated fats and trans-fatty acids while including monounsaturated fats (MUFAs) from avocados, olives and olive oil, nuts, seeds, and canola oil. Other good fats in the Mediterranean diet are omega-3 polyunsaturated fatty acids (PUFAs) that come primarily from flax seeds and fish. Also, unlike the traditional American diet, the Mediterranean diet is based on an abundance of plant foods, such as fresh fruits and vegetables, legumes, nuts, and whole grains.

In this chapter you discover the many benefits of following a Mediterranean diet, why MUFAs are good for you, where to find them, and the importance of eating these "good fats" to help you burn fat every day.

On the Mediterranean diet you'll learn how to make lean protein choices and understand why these foods can help you lose weight, trim belly fat, and look and feel your best. So take a culinary journey to the other side of the "pond" and get ready to enter the healthy world of Mediterranean cuisine.

The Mediterranean Miracle

Nutrition scientists first began looking at the Mediterranean diet shortly after World War II when they noticed people living around the Mediterranean Sea suffered fewer heart attacks than Northern Europeans and Americans. But, it wasn't until 20 years later when results from these studies showed the Mediterranean diet was protective against cardiovascular disease and lowered LDLs (bad cholesterol) that it became popular among health-care professionals.

WHAT'S NEW

Ancel Keys was the first scientist to demonstrate the positive health outcomes of the Med diet with his landmark Seven Countries Study. Published in 1970, this was the first study to establish a relationship between cardiovascular disease and saturated fat and cholesterol.

During the last 50 years, much scientific evidence has emerged to back up this diet's heart-healthy effects. There are also many newer findings that have shown the diet benefits more than just your heart. We now know the Med-style diet may also help reduce your risk of Type 2 diabetes, obesity, depression, metabolic syndrome, high blood pressure, and cancer of the breast, colon, pancreas, prostate, and endometrium.

Scientists have recently found a connection between the Mediterranean diet and brain function. Specifically, people who follow a Mediterranean diet and get regular exercise are nearly 40 percent less likely to develop Alzheimer's disease (AD) than those who don't eat this way and are sedentary. And, for those who already have AD, the Med diet may increase life expectancy by as much as four years.

Disease states aside, there are other pay offs, too. Eating the Mediterranean way can keep your brain young. As we age, our brains naturally begin to decline, resulting in "senior moments" such as forgetting where we put our keys or failing to remember someone's name. Although these are normal signs of aging, following a Mediterranean diet can slow down this effect. In fact, one study showed people who ate a more traditional Mediterranean diet had brains that functioned at a level several years younger than their chronological ages.

Part of the association with these brain benefits has to do with how much belly fat you have. People who follow a Mediterranean diet generally have smaller waistlines than those who don't and this makes a difference when it comes to brain health.

A California study looking at body fat and Alzheimer's disease in more than 8,700 men and women found the group with the most belly fat had nearly triple the risk of AD compared to those with the slimmest waistlines.

You're also more likely to keep your mind sharp if you stay fit and trim long-term. One French study found that subjects with a lower Body Mass Index (BMI) (i.e., smaller waist circumference) scored higher on cognitive performance tests than those who were heavier, regardless of age.

A Way of Living Lean—and Long

Although the Mediterranean diet is more likely to be touted as a healthy way of eating than a weight-loss regimen, it's easy to lose pounds on this diet, particularly if you are overweight. Several studies comparing low-fat diets to moderate fat (35 to 40 percent fat) Med-style diets, found those on the Med diet lost more weight than those on the low-fat diets. Furthermore they were more likely to keep the weight off over the long haul as well.

This makes sense considering people usually don't feel like they're on a "diet" when they start eating this way; rather, they're just making healthful food choices. Thus, they're more likely to stick to the Med plan than those on a lower fat (and less satisfying) diet.

Another factor has to do with the Med "diet" itself, which is not really a diet per se but a lifestyle—a lifestyle that includes leisurely meals (no eating in the car here), savoring meals with friends (eating is a social occasion to be shared with friends and family), and regular physical activity (usually in the form of walking after dinner).

How do these lifestyle factors keep you slim, trim, and healthy? First of all, eating in a social environment where people actually pay attention to their food helps you become a more mindful eater (see more about mindful eating in Chapter 10), which makes you more aware of how you're feeling, how much you are eating, and when you're feeling full.

This also means portion sizes tend to be smaller. Sometimes this is because there are several courses, and the fact that you are more conscious of what you eat, but more likely it has to do with the attitude about food. Europeans, especially, tend to value quality over quantity, thus smaller portions are not only accepted, but valued in this society.

Finally to eat Mediterranean is to savor and enjoy your food with people you care about. Thus a meal is a sit-down affair that can take anywhere from 30 minutes to several hours. Eating slowly not only gives you more time to taste and experience your food, it also gives your body more time to relax and respond to your meal. Studies comparing fast eaters to slow eaters found those people who ate slower had a higher concentration of the hormone that makes you feel full (leptin is the hormone that controls appetite), meaning your stomach has more time to send a satiety or fullness signal to your brain when you've had enough, thus preventing you from overeating.

GOOD MOVE

Chew your food, a lot. A Journal of the American Dietetic Association study comparing fast eaters to slow eaters reported that women who ate slowly, chewing each bite 20 to 30 times, felt fuller and ate 10 percent fewer calories than those women who ate fast.

Add up all these benefits and it's not surprising to find that people who eat (and live) like those in Mediterranean countries live longer and have a better quality of life than the general population, mainly because they have a lower incidence of most major chronic illness. According to a 2011 Dutch study, analyzing lifestyle components, eating a Mediterranean diet, not smoking, keeping your weight in the normal range, and getting regular physical activity means you could potentially live an extra 15 years for women and 8 years for men.

Recently, a British study looking at the components of the Med diet found that although all the elements of the diet contribute to good health, when it comes to a longer life some are more important than others. What were they? More vegetables, less meat, and of course, adding olive oil to food (best combined with vegetables).

Delicious Foods Packed with Nutrients

Healthy Mediterranean food consists of seafood, nuts, legumes, olives and olive oil, whole grains, fresh fruits and vegetables, moderate amounts of alcohol (mainly red wine), and relatively small amounts of red meat, chicken, and dairy. Thus, there is very little processed or packaged food in the diet. Consequently, this kind of fresh, whole, natural food is chock full of vitamins, minerals, antioxidants, and phytochemicals.

Sweets, although a regular part of the day in Italy, are generally bite-sized treats often eaten as a snack in the middle of the day. In other countries they are more often than not a special occasion treat—usually fresh fruit finishes out the meal.

Soft drinks, although becoming much more common, particularly among young people, are not part of the Mediterranean culture. Rather it's water, red wine, an occasional fruit juice, and tea or coffee.

Almost any lifestyle or kind of food can be adapted to fit this style of eating, meaning you don't have to be from the Mediterranean to eat Mediterranean-style food; American, Scandinavian, Russian, and Asian cuisine or just about any type of food can also work. The key is starting with whole, natural unprocessed foods and not fussing or fawning over them. Keep dishes simple with only a few ingredients, keep cooking techniques simple and easy, and season with fresh herbs and spices.

The Amazing Power of MUFAs

Much of the Mediterranean diet's healthy benefits are attributed to the copious use of olives and olive oil, the main source of fat in the diet. And, although olive oil is a nutritional powerhouse on its own, high in phenolic compounds, anti-inflammatory agents, and antioxidants, the fact that it is part of the family of monounsaturated fats, or MUFAs, is what put it in the nutritional spotlight.

RED FLAG

To lose belly fat, go easy on saturated fats found in whole milk, butter, cheese, and red meat. One small 2003 Australian study published in the *British Journal of Nutrition* looked at weight loss and fat mass on people following either a high saturated fat diet or a high monounsaturated fat diet and found that those on the MUFA-rich diet lost slightly more weight and fat mass compared to those on a high sat-fat diet, despite similar calorie levels and energy expenditure. One possible reason for this could be that your body is more likely to store saturated fat as fat, while MUFA is more likely to get utilized for energy.

During the last few years, research on MUFAs has been piling up fast. Originally touted as simply a good substitute for saturated fat for those concerned about heart disease, scientists soon learned that MUFAs did much more than that. Numerous studies showed MUFAs, themselves, could lower LDLs, total cholesterol, and triglyceride levels, without lowering HDLs (good cholesterol). Eventually scientists discovered that MUFAs protect against far more than cholesterol and heart disease.

Data now shows MUFAs can reduce your risk of Type 2 diabetes and insulin resistance, metabolic syndrome, breast cancer, inflammation, and high blood pressure.

When it comes to belly fat, MUFAs are more important than you think. Not only does a monounsaturated fat-rich diet help you lose weight, but even when weight remains unchanged, MUFAs redistribute body fat, pulling body fat out of the belly and moving it to other places like the legs. They also improve insulin sensitivity, which means cells are more likely to use the energy at hand. Carbohydrate-rich diets on the other hand, do just the opposite, upping abdominal fat and increasing insulin resistance.

What Is a MUFA?

All fats and oils are composed of medium or long chain fatty acids. These chains are a mixture of saturated, monounsaturated, and polyunsaturated fatty acids. Their classification is determined by the type of fatty acid that makes up the majority of the fatty acids.

Saturated fats are solid and waxy at room temperature and are primarily found in animal foods such as butter, red meat, and cheese with three exceptions—the plant foods coconut oil, palm and palm kernel oil, and cocoa butter. In the body, these solid saturated fats turn sticky and gummy, so they can easily stick to artery walls causing plaque to build up and increasing your risk of cardiovascular disease.

Unsaturated fats like MUFAs are liquid at room temperature and may turn semi solid in the refrigerator (think cloudy olive oil). Both MUFAs and PUFAs (polyunsaturated fats) are mainly found in plant foods. In the body, MUFAs and PUFAs are more likely to glide, flowing easily in the bloodstream. But MUFAs may have many extra-protective effects that PUFAs lack.

Where to Find MUFAs

MUFAs are naturally found in many nutrient-packed plant foods. Here are the best of the bunch:

- **Olive oil**—Although there are many good monounsaturated oils (peanut oil, canola oil, safflower oil, sesame seed oil, and nut oils), olive oil tops the list as the healthiest. About 80 percent of olive oil is made up of monounsaturated fatty acids. Extra virgin olive oil (EVOO), which is the least processed of the olive oils, is high in antioxidants, anti-inflammatory agents, and compounds that can lower LDLs and raise HDLs. In addition to protecting against heart disease, studies also suggest olive oil can reduce your risk of stroke, ulcerative colitis, breast cancer, obesity, and metabolic syndrome.

WHAT'S NEW

High-quality extra virgin olive oil contains oleocanthal, the compound that gives you a sting in the back of your throat after you swallow olive oil. Oleocanthal has been shown to protect against heart disease and dementia through its anti-inflammatory effects and is so potent that eating three or four tablespoons of extra virgin olive oil a day can have the same protective power as taking a daily baby aspirin. Although this amount is commonly consumed in the Mediterranean region, such large amounts of olive oil are not recommended here because they can add almost 500 calories to your daily diet.

- **Avocados**—Behind olive oil, avocados are the second richest source of mono-unsaturated fats in the diet. They're also high in fiber, vitamin E, vitamin K, folate, and potassium. Like olive oil, the MUFAs in avocados have been shown to fight heart disease. Avocados also have lutein and zeaxanthin, two compounds which protect eye health.

- **Nuts and nut butters**—Nuts are nutritional powerhouses loaded with fiber and many hard-to-get vitamins and minerals like vitamin E, selenium, zinc, copper, and manganese. Each one has unique health benefits that can protect you against many chronic diseases, but some pack extra nutritional punch. Almonds have the highest amounts of vitamin E, while walnuts have the most omega-3s of all nuts. Brazil nuts are highest in selenium, an anti-oxidant mineral that's been shown to be protective against breast cancer. Because nuts fill you up they also curb appetite, which is important for people who want to lose or even maintain weight. Be sure to practice portion control when eating nuts as some of the large containers of nuts can pack nearly 2,000 calories, and stick with unsalted ones to avoid water retention.

- **Seeds**—Pumpkin seeds, sunflower seeds, sesame seeds, and hemp seeds are all good sources of healthy monounsaturated fats. Like nuts, they are a good source of hard-to-get nutrients like magnesium, manganese, iron, calcium, copper, and zinc. They're also high in fiber, which helps us to feel satiated for longer.

- **Olives**—Olives are a staple in the Mediterranean regions and there are dozens to choose from. Aside from all the benefits of olive oil, olives give you fiber, vitamin E, iron, and copper.

Eat MUFAs Every Day

Considering all the benefits of monounsaturated fats it's no surprise that you should try to include some of these foods in your daily Flat Belly Diet. Eating them on a regular basis will not only help you lose weight and keep the weight you've already lost from creeping back on, they will also keep you satisfied and happy. Who doesn't want a little olive oil on their vegetables? Here are a few ways to eat MUFAs every day:

- Use olive oil as your primary cooking oil.

- Bring nuts with you when you're running errands so you can snack on them in-between meals.

- Keep a bowl of olives in the refrigerator within easy reach. All you need are three to five olives (depending on size) to get your benefits.

- Sprinkle seeds on your salads and vegetables.

RED FLAG

Don't *pour* on the olive oil. Although a little is good, a lot is not. Keep in mind that one tablespoon has 120 calories and 14 grams of pure fat.

What Protein Does for You

When most people think of protein they think of building and maintaining strong muscles—and that's true. But protein does much more than that. It keeps your immune system running; makes enzymes and hormones; is involved in tissue repair; builds cells that regularly break down, like your hair, nails, and skin; regulates fluid balance; transports nutrients; and is part of your genetic make-up. Proteins are vital for every function in your body including proper digestion.

Proteins are made up of amino acids. These 20 different amino acids are like building blocks that can be mixed and matched and strung together in millions of different ways to create the thousands of proteins our bodies need regularly.

During a meal that includes protein, fat, and carbohydrates, protein slows the rise in blood sugar that carbohydrates generally trigger. It also keeps us feeling full longer, which is why high protein diets have been shown to result in weight loss. The key is to choose lean protein that is low in saturated fat, such as chicken, turkey, or roast beef.

WHAT'S NEW

Your brain uses amino acids to transmit billions of instant messages to neurons every day. To keep these neurotransmitters functioning properly your brain needs a daily supply of high-quality protein.

How Much Protein You Really Need

If you deprive your body of protein, you'll be tired and dragging, your muscles will become weak, and you won't be able to concentrate (your brain, which needs a steady supply of amino acids, will be less sharp).

If you consume more protein than the body needs, your body will simply convert this protein to fat that likely will go straight to your belly. The U.S. Recommended Dietary Allowances suggest .8 grams protein per kilogram (kg) body weight. As you increase your physical activity, you'll need to up your intake to between 1.2 to 1.4 grams per kg per day. Keep in mind, however, that for healthy adults, protein should make up no more than 25 percent of total calories per day and as a minimum of no less than 15 percent of total calories per day.

GOOD MOVE

Calculating your protein needs is easy. Start by converting your weight from pounds to kilograms. For a 154-pound person, this is 154 lb/2.2 = 70 kg. Then multiply your weight in kg by 0.8 if you're not physically active. For our 70 kg person, that's 70 kg × 0.8 g/kg = 56 g protein per day. As you increase your physical activity, your protein needs will increase as well, so multiply your weight in kg by 1.2 and 1.4. For a 70 kg person, that's 70 kg × 1.2 g/kg = 84 g and 70 kg × 1.4 g/kg = 98 g protein per day.

High-quality lean protein (anywhere from 3 to 6 ounces of fish, chicken, or lean beef in one meal) is best. Just as important as what you eat is when you eat it. To get the most bang for your buck you should eat small amounts of protein throughout the day. Unfortunately, most Americans eat their protein all at once at dinner.

GOOD MOVE

In general try to aim for about 30 grams of protein in each meal. That's about a 4-ounce piece of steak, chicken, or fish, or 2 cups of black beans and brown rice topped with 1½ ounces of cheese.

Trim Belly Protein Sources

Protein is found in both plants and animals. Though the animal sources are most concentrated they are also the ones most likely to be high in saturated fat and total fat. So try to incorporate a mix of both plant and animal proteins in your diet—meaning add some vegetarian meals to your repertoire. Either way—plant or animal—be sure and choose lean, low fat, or "good" fat varieties. Here are a few to get you started.

Fish and Seafood

Fish and seafood are an excellent source of high-quality protein. They generally fall into two camps: lean fish and oily fish. Lean fish are shellfish like shrimp, crab, lobster, clams, and mussels, and white fish like tilapia, cod, and sole. Oily fish include salmon, trout, tuna, mackerel, herring, and sardines. Oily fish have a double benefit: first, they're high in protein, and second, they are a good source of *essential fatty acids (EFAs)*. EFAs are essential to life and include both omega-3 fatty acids and omega-6 fatty acids.

DEFINITION

Essential fatty acids (EFAs), like all "essential nutrients," are nutrients your body cannot make itself, so they must be obtained from the diet. EFAs are linoleic acid, known as an omega-6 fatty acid, and alpha linolenic acid, which is known as an omega-3 fatty acid.

In Paleolithic times, the ratio of omega-3 to omega-6 fatty acids was suspected to be somewhere around 1:1, thanks to a diet rich in fruit, vegetables, seafood, and wild game. Today, that ratio is more likely to be 15:1, higher in omega-6 fatty acids than omega-3 due to our extensive use of soybean and corn oil as well as newly imposed grain diets for livestock and inadequate amounts of fish in our diets.

Some scientists feel many of our modern health concerns can be attributed to this shift to a diet high in omega-6 and low in omega-3, and some people have had success reversing or improving disease states just by supplementing oils high in omega-3 fatty acids.

Rather than rely on a supplement, your best bet is to increase your intake of fish that live in colder waters and thus produce more oils for insulation like salmon, trout, anchovies, sardines, and fresh tuna. Other great sources of omega-3s are walnuts, flax, hemp, and omega-3 enriched eggs. Aim for including fish in at least one meal per day 4 to 5 times a week.

 RED FLAG

According to the FDA and EPA, pregnant women and small children should not eat swordfish, tilefish (golden snapper), king mackerel, and shark, because they may contain high levels of mercury. Eating a variety of other finfish and shellfish (up to 12 ounces per week) is recommended.

Lean Red Meat and Poultry

When it comes to red meat and poultry your best bet is to choose local grass-fed animals. Why? First, most of our livestock was naturally meant to eat grass. Feeding them a consistent diet of corn and grain upsets their natural balance and makes them more likely to get sick and need antibiotics or treatment. Second, grass-fed livestock is naturally leaner than corn fed, producing meat that is lower in total fat and thus, total calories.

Finally, not only is there less fat but the type of fat is different. Grass-fed beef is lower in saturated fat and higher in omega-3 fatty acids and CLA (conjugated linoleic acid), a good fat believed to have anti-cancer properties. Unlike conventionally fed beef, grass-fed beef is also high in vitamin E, a fat-soluble vitamin that has heart protective properties.

Beans and Lentils

Not only are beans and lentils a super-lean source of plant protein (they average about 14 grams of protein per 1 cup serving), they're also an excellent source of fiber, providing nearly half the recommended amount, 12 grams, in the same amount.

All this fiber along with protein is good news for belly fat. Bean eaters tend to be slimmer and have smaller waists than their nonbean eating counterparts. In one study, just an extra ½ cup of beans, amounting to about 10 grams of soluble fiber a day, was enough to reduce deep belly fat by nearly 4 percent in five years. Add in 30 minutes of activity a couple of times a week, and that number nearly doubles.

Nuts and Seeds

Adding nuts and seeds to your diet is another good way to bump up plant protein and keep you satisfied and feeling full until your next meal. Almonds, walnuts, hazelnuts, sunflower seeds, pumpkin seeds, and sesame seeds are all packed with protein, "good" monounsaturated and polyunsaturated fats, and a bevy of vitamins and minerals.

Remember to keep your serving size to one small handful, the equivalent of about one ounce, of nuts or two tablespoons of nut butter and you'll keep calories in check. To give you an idea of serving sizes, an ounce of nuts is equal to about 14 walnut halves or about 20 almonds or cashews.

The Least You Need to Know

- Following a Mediterranean diet lifestyle is the best way to slim down your belly, stave off chronic illness, and live a long, healthy life.
- Adding healthy monounsaturated fats to your diet in the forms of olive oil, olives, avocados, nuts, and seeds helps you lose weight, stay healthy, and prepare delicious, tasty foods you and your family will love.
- Protein is an important part of a healthy diet and should be included in every meal and snack throughout the day.
- Healthy protein foods include seafood, grass-fed beef and poultry, beans and lentils, and nuts and seeds.

Carbohydrates: Do's and Don'ts

In This Chapter

- It's all about the carbs
- Honing in on whole grains
- Facts about fiber
- Veggies and fruits you can count on

Carbohydrates come in many forms, some very healthy and some unhealthy. They include sugars, starches, and fiber.

Carbohydrates come from the sun. Well, actually, they come primarily from plants that make sugars using the energy of the sun. Plants make all sorts of carbohydrates, from the simplest sugars to large, complex fiber molecules. The primary function of carbohydrates is to provide energy for the body.

In Paleolithic times, carbohydrates were mainly eaten in the form of plant foods, but today, you're more likely to eat carbohydrates like cane sugar, high fructose corn syrup, and other added sugars. All this sugar has taken a toll on our health.

Nutritionists and obesity researchers are quickly reaching a consensus regarding the direct relationship between humans' drastic increase in sugar consumption during the last 150 years or so and our current epidemics of obesity and diabetes.

Although low-carbohydrate diets have been beneficial to some who want to lose weight, there seems to be an overly simplistic general "anti-carb" sentiment among many people. There are good carbs and there are bad carbs. In this chapter, we take a look at what carbohydrates are and what they do in the body—and which ones you should include in your everyday life to maximize your belly fat loss.

All Carbs Turn into Sugar Eventually

Digestion of carbohydrates begins in the mouth, by enzymes secreted in saliva. This makes sense from a Paleolithic perspective when you think of how rare and valuable these macronutrients are. When a hunter-gatherer found something sweet, she would eat as much as she could in response to the sense of calm, pleasure, and increased energy carbohydrates can provide. This is great if you're walking a lot and eating mostly veggies—but if almost everything you eat has sugar or corn syrup in it, you can easily end up consuming way too many calories.

Another reason for the high priority your body places on carbohydrate digestion is that your brain, unlike pretty much all other organs in your body, can only use glucose for fuel. Other structures, such as muscle and liver, can use fat and amino acids from proteins for energy. When carbohydrate intake is low and your protein intake is adequate, your brain is still well fed because your liver can produce plenty of glucose to keep it going, and excess body fat gets used up to fuel your muscles. This is the sort of physiology that you'll be shifting into on this belly fat loss program.

Because sugars are such small, simple molecules, your body absorbs them at lightning speed, driving your blood sugar way up at a pace you weren't built to be able to handle easily. In contrast, complex carbs are converted to simple sugars gradually, leading to a slower, less extreme uptick in blood sugar. When you get sugar in fruits and berries, you're giving your body great fuel in a way that it can use optimally.

Your body can store fat easily (obviously!), but it has a very limited ability to store carbohydrates. The liver and skeletal muscles can convert individual glucose molecules to a storage form called glycogen. The body's storage capacity for glycogen is only about 500 grams, so excess carb intake leads preferential use of carbohydrates for energy, leading the body to use little or no fat for energy. Over time, eating too many carbs leads to a condition where hardly any fat is burned—rather it's allowed to build up in the belly and elsewhere, causing overweight, obesity, and increased risk for disease.

It's All About Insulin

To fully understand how sugars and refined grains can increase your risk for belly fat, you have to take a quick look at insulin and how it works. You'll remember that the brain is totally dependent on sugar to function. Because of this, the rest of the body has a set of "brakes" on the surface of the cells that limit sugar uptake after every meal to assure that the brain stays well fed.

These "brakes" are insulin receptors; large particles made mostly of protein that sit on the surface of cells and regulate sugar's ability to enter. Insulin receptors are found mostly on liver and skeletal cells because these parts of the body are very active and metabolically busy. Well … skeletal muscle is active if you are active. If you're sedentary, your skeletal muscles get lazy. In Chapter 12, we take a close look at what being a couch potato does to your skeletal muscles and belly fat, and I hope that information will motivate you to get out there for your daily walk!

 RED FLAG

A diet high in refined carbohydrates not only leads to spikes in blood sugar and added abdominal fat, it also can lead to insulin resistance, elevated fat levels in the blood, lower HDL (the protective form of cholesterol), and elevated blood pressure—all significant risk factors for Type 2 diabetes and heart disease.

Back to insulin—it's a steroid hormone made and released by special cells in the pancreas. When you have a healthy, active lifestyle and good diet, every meal that contains at least some carbohydrate results in a gradual but significant rise in blood sugar. This triggers insulin release. Assuming you didn't eat too much, and you're somewhat active, insulin goes to your muscles and liver to allow glucose to enter, and blood sugar comes back down.

For a variety of reasons, the typical American diet with its huge load of simple carbs and bad fats tends to cause the pancreas to secrete abnormally large amounts of insulin after eating—and they tend to stay high between meals, too. Over time, as insulin levels remain high, its target cells grow tired of being stimulated, so they make fewer receptors and the receptors they do make are resistant to insulin's message—this is called insulin resistance—and this is the leading risk factor for Type 2 diabetes.

A primary goal of this flat-belly program is to give your pancreas and your insulin receptors a break by encouraging you to keep your carbs complex, fiber intake high, total carb intake per meal controlled, and your muscles moving. These simple steps will cause a dramatic drop in your blood insulin levels, protecting you against the likelihood of developing diabetes.

Simple vs. Complex Carbs

All carbohydrates can be classified as either simple or complex. A simple carbohydrate is one that can be digested and absorbed quickly and easily by the human body. Simple carbs tend to be either monosaccharides such as fructose from fruit, or disaccharides like lactose in milk and sucrose (table sugar).

Complex carbohydrates are larger molecules classified as either starch or fiber, depending on their size, structure, and digestibility. They're found in legumes, vegetables, and whole grains. Simple carbohydrates tend to provide only calories, but many foods containing complex carbs offer vitamins and minerals as well.

For optimal weight and health, carbohydrates should come almost exclusively in the form of complex carbohydrates such as fiber and starch. Our diet should have two to three times more fiber than what we typically eat today. Pre-agricultural humans had almost no intake of simple carbohydrates like sugars and refined flour at all. Many nutritional experts point to the drastic shift away from complex to simple carbohydrates as a major culprit in our epidemic of Type 2 diabetes and abdominal fat.

Impact of Carbohydrates on Belly Fat

As you've seen, simple carbohydrates set you up for a bigger belly. But not all carbs are bad, and they should stay in your diet. There are several ways that getting adequate amounts of complex carbs, especially fiber, in your diet can help get rid of belly fat:

- It adds bulk to any meal because it absorbs water in the intestine, giving an enhanced "full" feeling.

- High-fiber foods take more work and time to chew, which slows down food consumption and can lead to eating less.

- Fiber slows the absorption of sugar, leading to smaller blood sugar and insulin "spikes" after eating, which in turn reduces the body's tendency to store more energy as fat.

- Carbohydrates contain amino acids that travel to the brain and contribute to serotonin levels, which help your mood stay positive.

WHAT'S NEW

A recent study of obese people on a calorie-controlled diet found that those people who ate whole grains lost significantly more weight around the abdomen than those who ate the same amount of refined grains. The researchers speculated that this was because whole grains support healthier blood sugar levels, allowing fat to be used as fuel.

Get Complex Carbs from Grains, Veggies, and Fruit

Whole grains used to be a staple of the human diet. As people developed a taste for pastries and lighter breads, *refined* grains replaced them in almost everything. Refined grains also last longer than whole grains do. White flour, made mostly from refined wheat, is the basis of most of the cereals, breads, pastas, and snacks that Americans eat. The *process* removes the bran and the germ from the wheat kernel. Many experts believe that the loss of whole grains as a staple of the American diet is a major factor in the obesity and diabetes epidemics.

White flour is usually enriched with a few of the vitamins found in whole wheat, such as iron and four B vitamins. Unfortunately, enrichment cannot replace all of the many nutrients found in the bran and germ. Enriched white flour remains far inferior to whole-grain flour as a source of magnesium, zinc, B_6, and many other essential nutrients, making it almost completely without value as a source of fiber.

DEFINITION

Processed foods are foods that have been treated in some way to change their sensory, physical, or chemical properties. **Refining** is a type of processing in which the coarse parts of a food are removed.

Wheat bran is high in fiber and protein. Wheat germ is rich in essential fatty acids and numerous vitamins and minerals. When the bran and germ are removed, what's left behind is the core, which is practically all starch. Although starch is a complex carbohydrate, when it's eaten without any fiber it's easily and quickly broken down to simple sugars. Because of this, foods made with refined flour tend to trigger a rapid rise in blood sugar, followed by a big rise in insulin—which can lead to the formation of belly fat, especially when cortisol levels are also high.

Fiber: The Healthiest Carbohydrate

Fiber comes from plants and is made up of complex, nonstarch carbohydrates that aren't digestible in the small intestine. Because they aren't digested, when they arrive in the colon they're still whole, and available for the bacteria that live there to use them for fuel in a fermentation process. Fiber doesn't add calories to your diet, but it does provide important nutrients that are released when the bacteria break it down. The general recommendation for adequate fiber intake in adults is 14 grams for every 1,000 calories consumed per day. For a person on a 1,600 calorie diet, that amounts to about 22 or 23 grams. Unfortunately, most Americans only get about half that amount. The following table provides specific recommendations for people at all ages. Deficiencies in fiber are associated with constipation and other digestive problems, an increased risk of colon cancer, and heart disease.

Recommended Intake Levels for Fiber (Grams/Day)

Age (Year)	Male	Female
9–13	31	26
14–18	38	26
19–50	38	25
>50	30	21

The best sources of fiber are whole grains, legumes, vegetables, nuts, seeds, and fruits. (See Appendix C for a list of high-fiber foods.) Some doctors recommend fiber supplements to their patients, but it's really best to get all your fiber from food because of the valuable micronutrients and other compounds available from natural fiber sources.

The advantages of fiber are many, including prevention of hemorrhoids, constipation, and diverticulosis, and decreasing blood cholesterol levels. Another benefit of a high-fiber diet is its ability to suppress appetite. Several studies have shown that eating a high-fiber breakfast tends to lead to consuming less food and fewer calories at lunch time.

Soluble vs. Insoluble Fiber

Soluble fibers include pectin and gum. They're found inside plant cells, and released when eaten. They help moderate the speed with which you absorb the sugar in whole fruits because when you eat an intact fruit like an apple, you're getting the fiber along with the sugar, which slows your absorption of the sugar. During digestion of a whole fruit, these fibers absorb water and expand, which is why you tend to feel full after eating them. They help your body make bulkier and softer stool, which is easier and less stressful for your colon to pass. Soluble fibers also help to decrease cholesterol levels. Beans, dried peas, nuts, oats, blueberries, apples, and carrots are some of the fruits and vegetables that contain soluble fiber.

Insoluble fiber comes from the cell walls of plants. They include cellulose and lignin. These fibers tend to make your stool bulkier and speed up the movement of food through your digestive tract. This is thought to protect against colon cancer because it minimizes the time that any potentially harmful food contaminants are in contact with your intestinal tract. The best sources of insoluble fiber are carrots, apples, oats, peas, beans, citrus fruits, and barley.

With all the benefits of both types of fiber, it's clearly a good idea to get plenty of both. That's why this lifestyle plan has an emphasis on veggies, whole grains, and beans. After a few days on this program, you'll probably notice that your bowel movements are bulkier, more regular, and perhaps softer. That's a great sign—it means your body is getting a lot of benefit from your new eating habits!

Keeping Cholesterol in Check

Fiber, as it moves through the small intestine, has the capacity to absorb bile acids that are released into the digestive tract by the liver. These acids are produced in part from cholesterol, and if they aren't bound to fiber and excreted in stool, they can be re-absorbed into the liver. If the bile acids are consistently leaving the body, the liver needs to continually make more out of cholesterol, and this keeps levels in the body low.

The cholesterol the liver likes to use to make bile is found primarily in LDL particles which, as seen, are the among the most hazardous of blood lipids when levels are high. So fiber, by pulling bile salts out of the body in your stool, keeps your liver hopping, breaking down LDLs that could otherwise end up in the walls of your arteries making heart attack- and stroke-causing plaque.

The fiber in rolled oats is particularly talented at binding up and removing bile, which is produced and released by the liver to clear the body of excess fats and cholesterol. It's so good at this that the government allows foods like whole oats and barley to sport labels touting their ability to reduce the risk of heart disease. Pectin, a soluble fiber, is also a good bile salt binder, providing the benefit of lowered blood cholesterol.

Whole Grains = Good Carbs

You've already seen that eating whole instead of refined grains helps your blood cholesterol and the health of your colon. But there are even more reasons to choose unprocessed grains when it's time to eat. There's a large volume of research out there documenting the benefits of whole grains in the diet; eating a diet rich in whole grains ...

- decreases the risk of stroke by about $\frac{1}{3}$
- decreases the odds of developing Type 2 diabetes by about $\frac{1}{4}$
- reduces the incidence of heart disease by about $\frac{1}{4}$
- assists with long-term weight maintenance

What is meant by saying "whole grains?" Grain is, simply, the seed of a plant. As long as the grain is in its natural state when you cook and eat it, it's "whole." The process of refining wheat strips away both the germ and the bran layers, thus dramatically decreasing fiber content.

Whole grains are actually a pretty good source of protein, but the refining process removes about 25 percent of it. In addition, the unsaturated fat from the wheat germ is lost, and more than 17 key nutrients, including magnesium, selenium, copper, and manganese, are lost when the bran and germ are stripped away. These are essential minerals, protecting us against diabetes and heart disease.

WHAT'S NEW

A 2010 Tufts University study found that people who eat mostly whole grains had significantly smaller waist circumferences than those eating white bread and flour—while consuming roughly the same number of calories. In fact, the people who ate primarily refined grains had about 20 percent more belly fat than those who ate them very rarely.

The U.S. government's dietary guidelines call for eating at least half of the grains in your diet as whole grains, amounting to three to five servings a day. Many nutrition experts feel that's not enough and recommend trying to make at least ¾ of your grain intake whole. Unfortunately, the average American eats less than one serving of whole grains a day—and a whopping 40 percent never eat them at all.

Most studies of the benefits of whole grains have focused on oats, barley, quinoa, wheat, rice, corn, millet, and buckwheat. A serving of whole grains is generally ½ cup cooked grain, pasta, or oatmeal; one slice of whole-grain bread; or 1 cup of 100 percent whole-grain cold cereal. When you're shopping, don't be taken in by labels such as "multigrain," "cracked wheat," or "stone ground." None of these claims require the product to be made entirely of whole grains. Check the label. A whole-grain product will have the word "whole" in its description, such as "whole-wheat flour," and ideally, it will come first on the ingredient list, indicating that it's the most plentiful ingredient.

GOOD MOVE

Millions of people can't eat gluten, a protein found not only in wheat but also in barley, rye, spelt, kamut, and triticale. If you're one of them, you don't have to avoid grains altogether! There's a wide variety of gluten-free grains you can enjoy, including amaranth, corn, millet, quinoa (my personal favorite), rice, wild rice, and sorghum. Give some of these other grains a try and you'll be able to eat grain without a belly ache.

So what makes whole grains so great? You've already seen that they're very high in fiber and minerals that are essential for good health. They're also chock full of vitamins, especially the B vitamins that participate in a wide variety of vital cellular functions like DNA repair. Many of the chemicals plants make to protect themselves against infection and parasites are good for you, too. There's a dizzying array of these molecules in a single grain seed, and studies of their health benefits abound. The whole grains you eat are good food for the beneficial bacteria living in your colon, too. These helpful bacteria flourish when you eat enough whole-grain food, making them hardy defenders against other microbes that can cause disease.

All the mechanisms for the marvelous effects of grains haven't been worked out, but some have, including these:

- Fiber grabs water and makes food bulkier and more satisfying, reducing appetite.

- Whole grains have a blunting effect on the blood sugar and insulin rise that occurs after a meal, helping prevent the development of insulin resistance.

- Some grains cause changes in the levels of hormones made by the digestive tract—these hormones travel to the brain and suppress appetite.

Veggies Are Vital for Health

The USDA recommends that all adults eat between 5 and 13 servings of vegetables per day. A serving is defined as ½ cup of cooked or raw veggies, except greens like lettuce or spinach. For these leafy vegetables, a serving is 1 cup. There are many reasons why you should meet, if not exceed, the USDA's guidelines:

- Vegetables provide maximal nutrition per calorie.

- Vegetables are high in fiber.

- Vegetables contain phytochemicals that help protect your body from damage to your cells by carcinogens and other toxins.

- Vegetables are bulky, with a high water content, so you can eat until you're full without taking in many calories.

Despite all these benefits, vegetables are often overlooked at meal and snack times. It's estimated that the average American adult barely meets half the recommended intake of vegetables every day.

Veggies Are Loaded with Filling Fiber

Although legumes are the foods highest in fiber, vegetables are no slouches in that regard. It's not always obvious from a veggie's texture how much fiber a serving contains, however. Even though a carrot may seem crunchy and fibrous, it provides only 1.7 grams of fiber, compared with a whopping 8.8 grams found in a cup of cooked peas. In addition to Appendix C, which provides the fiber content of a limited selection of foods, you'll find good websites that provide the fiber content of a variety of different fruits and vegetables in Appendix B.

 GOOD MOVE

So much of what is good for us about vegetables is what we cannot digest or absorb. The fiber, both soluble and insoluble, passes through us, keeping us feeling full, providing food for healthy bacteria, removing excess cholesterol, and providing bulk for our stool. All of which are important for staying healthy and feeling good.

Phytonutrients, Antioxidants, and Water

There are many theories about what the perfect diet is for the human body, and there certainly isn't a full consensus among nutritionists on every point. But one point everyone seems to agree on is that we desperately need to increase our intake of fruits and vegetables. In practically every single study of the effects of diet on the incidence and severity of obesity, heart disease, and cancer, it's been found that all of these poor health outcomes are lowest in people who consume the most fruits and vegetables every day. We know this is due in part to the high fiber content of these foods, especially vegetables and berries. We also know that there are hundreds if not thousands of protective chemicals in these foods, called phytochemicals, which play specific roles in protecting our cells and organs from damage. Sadly, only about 16 percent of adults eat the 5 servings of fruits and vegetables per day recommended by the government.

"Phyto" refers to plants, and *phytonutrients* are molecules made by plants that benefit them and us. These chemicals include carotenoids, flavonoids, and other organic compounds. The carotenoids include the pigments that make fruits and vegetables red, orange, and yellow. Foods high in carotenoids have been found to be protective against certain cancers and heart disease, as well as macular degeneration. Some of the best sources of carotenoids are carrots, tomatoes, and citrus fruits.

> **DEFINITION**
>
> **Phytonutrients** is a broad term that refers to a large number of compounds pro-
> duced by plants that have been found to be beneficial to human health. Some
> important phytonutrients are carotenoids, one of which is lycopene, a bright red
> pigment found in tomatoes and other red fruits.

There are dozens, if not hundreds, of different phytonutrients in fruits and vegetables. A great deal of research has been done on the benefits of these molecules and
these benefits include …

- Antioxidant activity

- Enhanced immune function

- Causing cancer cells to die

- Helping the liver detoxify carcinogens

The average American consumes about three servings of vegetables every day.
Unfortunately, dark green vegetables and highly pigmented red and yellow vegetables
account for only a small portion of those eaten. When you are choosing vegetables to
eat, you'll get the best nutritional value for your money and efforts if you always go
for the most colorful choice. That means choosing romaine lettuce instead of iceberg,
broccoli instead of cauliflower, and making sure to include citrus fruits two or three
times a week.

Many people have the misconception that vital nutrients are destroyed when fruits
and vegetables are cooked. There are also people who believe that microwaving
destroys nutrients in food as well. A recent study of the effects of a variety of different methods of cooking on the antioxidants levels in food proved these assumptions
wrong.

According to the study, microwaving and steaming actually make some phytonutrients and antioxidants more available for absorption in the human digestive tract. So
while salads and raw fruits and vegetables are healthy and good for you and should be
eaten every day, you don't have to worry about losing the benefits of eating fruits and
vegetables if you prefer to cook them.

The Super Seven Vegetables for Health

As you've seen, vegetables provide a great variety of benefits to your health when you include them in your diet. Though all of them are healthy, some veggies emerge as nutritional all-stars, providing lots of fiber, phytonutrients, and vitamins when compared to others. Here is a list of veggies to add to your diet as often as possible to maximize your diet's health-boosting and belly flattening power:

- Cruciferous vegetables, including broccoli, cauliflower, Brussels sprouts, arugula, artichoke, and bok choy.

- Dark leafy greens such as romaine lettuce, kale, spinach, and the chards. These are versatile and packed with fiber and phytonutrients.

- Yams, sweet potatoes, and other orange foods—avoid peeling them to get the most fiber.

- Bell peppers in all colors are especially rich in vitamin C.

- Legumes are great sources of fiber and protein.

- Squash and pumpkin.

- Garlic and onions, including leeks, shallots, chives, and scallions.

Fresh vs. Frozen

Fresh vegetables are lovely—the colors, smells, and textures are enough to stimulate anyone's appetite. But many people think they don't have time to buy, prepare, and cook fresh veggies. There are lots of ways to make this whole process more efficient and quick, like shopping and chopping on one or two days a week and keeping prepped veggies in the fridge until they're used in a meal or recipe. If you're resistant to this, there's still no excuse not to eat your vegetables.

GOOD MOVE

Next to fresh, frozen fruits and vegetables are nearly as high in phytonutrients. Because frozen produce is frozen right at the farm, usually at the peak of freshness, sometimes frozen food is actually better nutritionally than fresh produce, which is usually not picked ripe and may sit around in your refrigerator or on the shelf for a week or more.

Frozen and canned fruits and veggies have just as much fiber as fresh ones do, and they also retain most of their micronutrients. Dried and crushed veggies and fruits have been found to be depleted in their fiber's ability to absorb water, however, and aren't recommended in your flat-belly lifestyle.

What About Fruit?

Fruits are delightful, sweet, nutritious foods that are part of any healthy diet. In the flat-belly plan, however, you'll be emphasizing vegetables over fruits to avoid taking in too much fructose. Another reason for limiting fruits is that you're working on retraining your palate to appreciate foods that aren't so sweet, to help cut down on sugar preferences and cravings. As you get closer to your weight and waist goal, you can bring more fruits into your daily diet.

With that said, there is one type of fruit you want to make sure you get enough of and that's berries. Berries play a big role in your flat-belly program because they pack a whollop of fiber and, because of this, they have the least effect on your blood sugar of all the fruits. Take raspberries for example. Although a cup of these little beauties has 14.7 grams of carbohydrate, 8 grams of them are fiber. That means that you're only getting about 6.7 grams of fructose and other simpler carbs per serving. In addition, their dark, intense color is a signal that they're well armed with phytonutrients that fight cancer and support immunity.

Several berries have emerged as powerful immune boosters, including the huckleberry and the acai berry. Research on these and other berries has shown that of all the fruits, berries are probably the most beneficial for health—and for weight loss. They may cost a little more than other fruits, but pound for pound, you're getting some premium nutritional and weight-loss support when you buy and eat them.

The Least You Need to Know

- Carbohydrates come primarily from plants and range from simple sugars to fiber.
- Simple carbs are digested and absorbed more quickly than complex carbs, and cause a more drastic insulin response.

- Fiber helps with weight loss by adding bulk to your diet and absorbing cholesterol-containing bile acids.

- Vegetables are a great source of fiber, vitamins, and other phytonutrients that support health and weight loss.

- Fruits, although a great source of fiber and phytonutrients, should be eaten sparingly to avoid possible blood sugar surges. Save them for daily snacks and choose high-fiber fruits like apples and citrus.

Drinks and Your Belly

In This Chapter

- Why you should wet your whistle with water
- How to shed the sugary drinks
- How to get energized with coffee and tea
- Why you don't need to be a teetotaler

What you drink and how much you drink can make or break your Flat Belly Diet. It can also mean the difference between a slim, trim tummy and an oversized pot belly. Quench your thirst with water and you can curb your appetite, flush out toxins, and stay energized throughout the day. Choose processed sugar-sweetened beverages instead and you're likely to get a bigger belly, bloated stomach, extra calories you don't need, and an increased risk for chronic illnesses like heart disease, stroke, diabetes, and obesity.

And, water isn't your only option either. Coffee drinkers will be happy to know that you don't have to give up your favorite beverage to have a lean waist, but you do have to keep your habit under control to get the best possible health benefits from this popular elixir. Read on to see how you can do this.

Alcoholic drinks also have their place, so if you're a wine, beer, or liquor drinker never fear—you can still enjoy a glass or two a day as long as you don't overdo it.

In the following pages you'll learn why liquid calories can be more dangerous to your health than eating too much food, which drinks you should drink and which ones to avoid, plus some belly beverage tips to keep you hydrated and healthy throughout the day.

The Wonders of Water

Of all the nutrients in our diet, water is the most important. Although you can live for weeks without food, you can only survive but a few days without water. That's because water is essential to all the life processes that go on in to your body. It is the medium through which you transport oxygen, red blood cells, vitamins and minerals, antibodies, enzymes, and hormones throughout the body. It eliminates wastes and toxins and it is involved in every reaction that builds up and breaks down cells. Water is required for digestion and absorption, brain function, muscle contractions, nerve transmission, and controlling body temperature.

> **WHAT'S NEW**
>
> Did you know that more than 60 percent of your body composition is made up of water? Much of it is in the form of blood, which is more than 80 percent water.

More than just keeping these basic functions moving is the way water affects how you feel. Staying hydrated can keep you feeling energized, relaxed, happy, and satisfied, making your stomach feel full.

For most people, good hydration means drinking six to eight 8-ounce glasses of water per day. Your daily water needs will vary with the temperature (you need more when it's hot) and activity levels. A good way to know if you're drinking enough is by checking the color of your urine. If it's light yellow, you're getting enough water.

Water as a Stress Reliever

Have you ever felt lightheaded, dizzy, or headachy, then took a drink of water only to have your symptoms immediately disappear?

Not getting enough water does more than just make you feel tired and fatigued. It stresses your entire body, including your heart and your mind.

Your brain is composed of 70 to 80 percent water, so when you don't drink enough water it shows. Your brain becomes stressed and has to work harder to perform the same tasks. Lack of water also effectively puts you in a bad mood, resulting in irritability and loss of concentration. These two things—feeling stressed and in a bad mood—can lead to poor food choices and overeating. The solution is to pay attention to your water intake and sip water throughout the day. It doesn't take much to slip into a dehydration state; when you're thirsty it's already too late.

Take a Drink Before You Eat

If not getting enough water could lead to eating too much, can getting enough (but not too much) mean you could actually eat less? Researchers think so. According to a 2010 study presented at the American Chemical Society in Boston, middle aged and older people who drink two cups of water before eating a meal ate 75 to 90 fewer calories than their non-water-drinking counterparts. Consequently, during a 12-week period, the water-drinking dieters lost more weight (nearly 5 pounds more) than the people who didn't drink water. Plus they kept it off after a year.

Why? Water makes you feel full, thus curbing your appetite. With zero calories it is also the ideal replacement for sugary, high-calorie drinks.

GOOD MOVE

Next time you want a drink of water, be sure to grab an icy cold one. Not only does it taste better, but your body has to work harder to warm it up, burning more calories and amping up your metabolism.

Sweetened Beverages: Liquid Candy

Look around and you'll see people drinking sodas morning, noon, and night. Given the popularity of these drinks it's no surprise that when it comes to U.S. beverage consumption, soft drinks now rank number one, beating out milk, juice, and water, even among children. Number two and three in line are no better—sugary energy drinks and sports drinks. But all these sweet beverages come with a price.

Liquid calories now make up about 22 percent of our total calorie intake, almost double of what it was in 1965. That's an extra 400 or more calories a day just from drinks, and most of these calories are in the form of high fructose corn syrup. In fact, half of our 22 teaspoons of added sugars a day comes from liquids.

The problem with this is that people don't compensate for these extra calories by eating less solid food. This is particularly obvious when people drink high-calorie drinks throughout the day. Generally, they eat the same amount of food whether they drank 2 cups of water or 2 cups of soda. The reason for this harkens back to our cavemen days when water was the only thing available. If man got filled up on no-calorie water, he wouldn't survive very long.

The second problem relates to the sugary drink itself. There's evidence that sugar or high fructose corn syrup (HFCS) consumed in liquid form does more harm to the body than sugars in food. This may be because these drinks are absorbed quickly, spiking blood sugar and insulin levels and disrupting blood lipid levels. They also go straight to your belly, raising your risk of diabetes, metabolic syndrome, and high blood pressure.

Worse yet is the fact that some studies show sugary drinks may even make you hungrier, causing you to eat more food than if you didn't drink these beverages.

WHAT'S NEW

One 12-ounce can of cola contains about 10 teaspoons of sugar (40 grams). A tall Starbucks Frappuccino has around 8 teaspoons of sugar.

Sans the Soda for Your Heart and Your Bones

Aside from the fact that soft drinks are empty calories, with no nutritional value and often replace healthier drinks like low-fat milk, is the news that soft drinks could be harmful to your heart. Just two soft drinks a day could increase a woman's risk of having a heart attack by 20 percent. This data was so strong that the American Heart Association recently advised all Americans to cut back on foods and drinks with added sugars (i.e., soft drinks), recommending no more than 6 teaspoons for women and 9 teaspoons for men. See the AHA new sugar guidelines at www.americanheart. org.

Soft drinks, and particularly colas, have also been associated with lower bone mineral density in women, related to losing more calcium in the urine than people who don't drink soda. Other research has linked soda with the rising incidence of gout and pancreatic cancer.

But, if you think you're safe because you're drinking diet soft drinks, think again. There is much controversy surrounding artificial sweeteners and the jury is still out as to whether they are safe or not. Like regular sodas, diet soft drinks keep you craving sweet drinks (and foods) and may even make you eat more food. Furthermore, many people who drink diet sodas often make unhealthy food choices as a reward for choosing a "diet" drink. Don't fall into this trap.

What About Fruit Juices?

Although they seem healthy, fruit juices are only minimally better for you than soda. That's because not all fruit juices contain the same type and amount of sugar. They all contain fructose, but the ratio of fructose to glucose varies from juice to juice. Some drinks can contain more sugar than soda, and because we don't compensate for the extra calories, it's easy to eat more and end up gaining weight rather than losing it.

So while fruit is a great vehicle for fiber and wonderful phytonutrients, juice, on the other hand, is a risky proposition when you're trying to lose weight, especially for children.

In kids the fructose in sugary drinks may cause fat cells in the abdomen to develop sooner and in greater numbers. This can set a child up for a lifetime of battling belly fat. As if that weren't bad enough, in lab research, fructose makes fat cells less responsive to insulin. This can lead to Type 2 diabetes, currently an epidemic among children in the United States.

To keep your blood sugar and insulin levels at a minimum and stable, you should avoid drinking fruit juice altogether while you're actively losing belly fat.

After that, however, always choose a calorie-controlled portion of 100 percent fruit juice (about 8 ounces a day) with no added sugars or artificial sweeteners. The upside is you can get a good dose of vitamins, minerals, and other phytochemicals from the fruit, but the downside is that juices contain very little fiber, and therefore this can have a jarring effect on blood sugar. So if you're going to drink juice, it's a good idea to stick to citrus juices like orange juice, for their very high content of vitamin C, or the dark red juices like grape, acai, or pomegranate for their high antioxidant content.

Your best bet for watching calories: dilute fruit juice by 50 percent with half water or seltzer. This reduces out the calories, while still quenching thirst.

Fruit Drinks Are Not Better

Juice is a popular drink among kids and adults alike. Unfortunately, many drinks on the market that appear to be juice are actually fruit "drinks." Fruit "drinks" contain very little actual juice, usually only 10 percent, and loads of sugar often in the form of HFCS. The only way to be sure you're drinking fruit juice is to squeeze it yourself or look for "100 percent fruit juice" on the label.

The one exception to this rule is cranberry juice, which is so tart and so acidic it's rarely sold without some type of sugar added to it (though you can find unsweetened varieties online). For this juice, look for low-sugar brands.

RED FLAG

Beware of labels that tout "low-sugar," "reduced sugar," or "low-calorie" on the label. Many times these products use artificial sweeteners to retain sweetness without the calories. Read the label to know for sure.

A Case for Caffeine

Together, coffee and tea are the two most widely consumed beverages in the world. What makes them so special? Two things: caffeine, which keeps you alert and energetic, and phytochemicals such as antioxidants and polyphenols that support good health by protecting your cells from stress and premature aging. The former stimulates the central nervous system, increasing alertness and boosting energy.

The question is, can caffeine affect weight loss and particularly belly fat? Yes and no. In the short-term caffeine speeds up metabolism and suppresses appetite, which leads to a slight increase in burning calories. For people who aren't used to drinking caffeinated beverages, caffeine can also result in weight loss through water loss. This diuretic effect doesn't happen with regular caffeine drinkers.

On the other hand, caffeine raises levels of our stress hormone cortisol, which can lead to weight gain. It also temporarily elevates blood pressure.

But, perhaps the most interesting aspect of caffeine involves its role in physical activity. We've known for years that small amounts of caffeine can improve endurance and performance in athletes. But, even for people who aren't athletes, one cup of coffee containing about 100 to 200 milligrams of caffeine an hour or so before a workout will give you a jolt, allowing you to work out longer and better.

This is one case, however, where more isn't better. In fact, too much coffee (more than four cups) can actually hinder your performance in the gym, causing heart palpitations, shakiness, and the jitters. It can also foster a physical dependence and lead to problems sleeping.

Coffee Perks

After many years of getting a bad rap, coffee has finally shaken its image as an "unhealthy" habit, vindicated by a parade of research showing that drinking java can guard us against heart disease, gallstones, kidney stones, gout, and various cancers including liver, colon, prostate, and certain breast cancers.

These benefits extend to the brain as well, as regular coffee drinkers have been shown to have lower rates of Alzheimer's disease and Parkinson's disease. There is even some evidence that coffee may slow age-related declines in memory and verbal recall.

And, according to the American Diabetes Association, regularly drinking a few cups of brewed coffee can significantly reduce your chances of getting Type 2 diabetes, by as much as 60 percent. Even people with diabetes can enjoy a cup of joe—sans the sugar—as long as it doesn't disrupt their blood sugar levels.

Caffeine may be responsible for some of these advantages, but most likely it's the hundreds of complex phytochemicals unique to this brewed beverage that have the biggest impact, many of which are antioxidants. Although not as nutritious as fruits and vegetables, coffee has proven to be the single greatest source of antioxidants in the U.S. diet, simply because we drink so much of it. The average American drinks two cups a day.

But, if you aren't a coffee drinker this isn't a license to start, and if you are a regular coffee drinker don't up your intake—on the Flat Belly Diet we recommend no more than 2 to 3 cups a day and no coffee except decaf after noon. This is because caffeine can stay in your system for 8 hours or longer, disturbing your sleep. Other negative side affects, particularly in sensitive individuals, include migraines, GI problems, heart palpitations, and interaction with medications.

Furthermore, although most of the coffee tested in studies was black without sugar or milk, the specialty coffee trend that swept the country and introduced the younger generation to the pleasures of coffee prides itself on serving high-calorie, flavored concoctions loaded with fat, sugar, and salt, such as a 16 ounce Starbucks White Chocolate Mocha that's packed with 500 calories. Instead, choose plain black coffee like Café Americano and put your own sugar, honey, or sweetener in it (if at all) and low-fat or nonfat milk. For an interesting twist, try adding soy or nut milks, like almond milk for an almond-flavored coffee.

More Tea, Please

Like coffee, tea contains a wealth of beneficial phytochemicals known for their anti-inflammatory, anti-carcinogenic, and anti-plaque-forming qualities. Indeed tea, especially green, has similar protective properties—defending against heart disease, cancer, diabetes, and brain decline—with fewer of coffee's negative side effects. It's also a beverage that's been around for thousands of years. Make sure you switch to herbal or decaffeinated green tea for late afternoon and evening drinking.

When it comes to losing belly fat, however, unsweetened brewed tea—black, oolong, or green—ranks up there with water as one of your top picks. Not only do these contain zero calories, meaning they're ideal for replacing sugary drinks, and come in a variety of flavors and styles to keep you feeling satisfied, but they also contain certain compounds that may help you lose weight. These compounds are called catechins, a phytochemical specific to tea (all types), and are particularly potent in green tea. A review of more than a dozen studies looking at green tea showed a modest reduction in BMI, body weight, and waist circumference independent of other factors. Recently, white tea has shown these same properties.

If you're looking to curb your appetite by increasing your fluid intake, tea—all kinds—is a good way to do it. Herbal teas, although not technically "teas" because they do not come from the tea plant camellia sinensis, do the same and have their own health benefits. Here you'll find mate, chamomile, rooibos, hibiscus, peppermint, chicory, and dozens more. Many times you'll find these herbs combined with black, green, or oolong tea to give a double dose of good-for-you phytochemicals. All in all, regularly drinking tea is a good habit to have.

WHAT'S NEW

The newest theme among tea manufacturers is "dessert" in a cup. These are herbal or regular teas infused with natural flavors like chocolate, coconut, vanilla, cinnamon, or ginger. With zero calories and all-natural ingredients, these are a good choice for the more adventurous tea drinker.

Toast to Your Health

Just because you want to live a healthy lifestyle and lose weight doesn't mean you have to give up drinking wine, beer, or liquor. On the contrary, those who enjoy imbibing from time to time may actually have an edge over nondrinkers when it comes to heart disease. That's because moderate alcohol consumption, one drink a day for a woman and two drinks a day for a man, can lower your risk of stroke, heart attack, and mortality related to cardiovascular disease.

And, it doesn't matter what type of drink either. While most research has focused on the benefits of red wine, thanks to the popularity of the Mediterranean diet, scientists have seen positive effects from beer and liquor.

GOOD MOVE

A drink is defined as 12 ounces of beer, 5 ounces of wine, or 1.5 ounces of 80-proof distilled spirits.

But alcohol may not benefit everyone who drinks. Even moderate drinking can increase the risk of breast cancer for some women. Luckily, there is a way to diminish this effect. Add more B vitamins to your diet, specifically folate, vitamin B_6, and B_{12}. Check with your doctor to find out more about this.

Remember, too, that calories from alcohol can rack up fast. One glass of wine can bump your daily quota more than 100 calories, so be sure and take this into consideration when trying to lose weight.

Even the healthiest beverages can turn bad if loaded up with sugar, artificial sweeteners, and/or fake flavorings. If you're not sure whether you can go without that sweet drink or second glass of wine, make your changes in small steps. Rather than go cold turkey, reduce the sugar in your coffee or tea by half first, then when you get accustomed to this you can cut it altogether. Dilute sweet drinks with water and think about spritzing your wine with seltzer instead of drinking it straight. For other alcoholic drinks, load up on ice cubes—you'll keep it cold and make it last longer. Keep a bottle of water on your desk as a reminder to sip it throughout the day. The water will fill you up, keep you hydrated, and energize your body.

The Least You Need to Know

- Drinking at least eight glasses of water a day will help you curb hunger, stay hydrated, and feel energized. Your urine should be light yellow in color as a good indicator that you are well hydrated.
- Remove or strictly limit sodas, fruit juices, and fruit drinks high in concentrated sugar and calories from your diet. They are more likely to add weight around your middle.
- Coffee and tea are high in beneficial antioxidants, and if drank with only small amounts of sugar and milk should be included on the Flat Belly Diet.
- If you currently don't drink alcohol, don't start. But, if you do, drink only in moderation.

Getting a Handle on Stress

Of all the factors that affect belly fat, stress has got to be one of the biggest. Not only does stress cause us to overeat, but it can also put on the pounds especially around the middle, not to mention do a number on our health. Here you'll get plenty of tips and tricks on how to "de-stress" your life and get yourself into emotional balance, including three pathways to a calmer, leaner self. Because stress often influences what, when, and how much you eat, getting stress under control can do wonders for your diet and your body.

Calm Mind, Lean Body

In This Chapter

- Stress isn't what happens to you, it's how you see it
- Stress leads to bad moods that often result from faulty thinking
- Good coping keeps you healthy and lean

Losing belly fat is about more than what you eat and how much physical activity and exercise you get. As we've seen, the cortisol released during acute and chronic stress is a major contributor to that big belly. In the next chapter, we're going to offer you some effective ways to keep yourself cool and collected, even during stressful times. In this chapter, we take a look at how life events, thoughts, and feelings affect you—and how you can avoid letting them be hazardous to your health.

Stress Is About Perception

We all know people who seem to ride out the storms of life with a remarkable sense of calm and capability. You can probably also think of people who "freak out" at the slightest setback, and really fall apart when things get tough. In his book *The Healing Mind*, Dr. Paul Martin describes stress as "the state arising when the individual perceives that the demands placed on them exceed (or threaten to exceed) their capacity to cope, and therefore threaten their wellbeing."

This is a great definition of stress, because it acknowledges the central role of perception as the trigger for the brain and the body's physiological changes that we call the stress response, described in Chapter 3. The stress response, except in extreme circumstances, doesn't arise because of what happens to us, but rather because of what we think about what happens to us. This is a critical distinction, and the core principle of effective stress management.

Challenge or Threat?

For most of us, everyday life is relatively safe and predictable—but unpleasant, frightening, frustrating, and sad things happen all the time. Divorce, unemployment, money problems, death of family members—these events are very disruptive and upsetting to just about anyone. In the early days of stress research, it was thought that the best way to measure a person's health risk related to stress was to simply add up the number of big life events they'd experienced in the last year. The greater the number of events, the more likely a person would be suffering the effects of stress, it was thought.

WHAT'S NEW

Dozens of studies have shown that people who perceive their jobs as stressful and overwhelming have significantly higher levels of cortisol than people in the same jobs who see them as challenging and manageable.

Over time, it became clear that counting life events doesn't reliably predict a person's cortisol level, belly fat, blood pressure, or other markers of chronic stress. It turns out that it's a person's perception of how stressful life is that matters, which is why we ask you to complete the Perceived Stress Scale in Chapter 15. What stress researchers have found is that physical stress states arise in response to any perception of threat. So it's possible for a person living in the most luxurious and seemingly trouble-free environment to be stressed out. It's also possible for a person living in difficult circumstances to view her struggles as a challenge with an opportunity for growth and to thrive.

Stressful Thoughts

In cognitive psychology, the goal is to help a person identify faulty patterns of thinking that are causing distress. It's helpful to uncover and examine these often irrational assumptions and attributions so they can be challenged and, in many cases, defused. Here are some common habits of mind that can create stress:

- **Catastrophizing:** People with this tendency often, if not always, take every little problem to its worst possible outcome, and respond to that instead of what's really happening.

- **Assumed omnipotence:** This is the assumption that one can control the uncontrollable. Many people get upset about things they see on the news, the outcome of sporting events, and the opinions and behaviors of other people—among other things.

- **Useless worry:** Threat perceptions can arise in response to what's happening in the moment, but even more often they arise in response to memories of past upsets and worries about future problems. Good stress management requires being able to put things into perspective by letting go of past mistakes and setbacks, and learning to stop worrying about what might happen in the future.

- **Overpersonalizing:** This type of thinking leads a person to feel overly responsible for other people's moods and behaviors, leading to feelings of self-consciousness and anxiety in social situations.

What Is Coping?

Coping is what you do in response to any perception that things are "just too much," or any thought or event that you perceive as negative—a potential threat to the survival, health, happiness, independence, or self-esteem of yourself or someone you care about. Coping takes the form of thoughts and behaviors, and it's done in an effort to lessen the negative effects of what's bothering you.

There are two major types of coping: *emotional regulation* and *problem management*. To be good at buffering stress, you need to be skilled at both. Emotional regulation is anything you tell yourself or do in order to feel less angry, scared, or sad about a negative situation. Problem management usually involves taking action to solve an issue or prevent it from happening in the future.

DEFINITION

Emotional regulation is the process of recognizing, accepting, and appropriately modulating or expressing one's emotional responses to life events and one's thoughts. **Problem management** is the type of coping behavior that is directed at changing a stressful situation by addressing root causes and predisposing conditions.

Coping strategies are usually learned over the course of your lifetime, and they tend to become habitual—that is, you often don't stop and examine the things you think and do when you feel threatened. Most of us simply react. Skillful coping can lead to positive, healthy outcomes in the face of life's challenges. Poor coping often leads to more stress, poor health, and general unhappiness.

Unhealthy Coping

In general, unhealthy coping responses tend to involve avoiding problems, seeking quick fixes, and "numbing out." Unhealthy types of emotional regulation include overeating; eating fatty, sugary foods; and watching television. Many people turn to food to feel better when they're stressed, as we saw in Chapter 3. Unfortunately, comfort food's effects are short-lived—but their impact on your belly and your health can last a lifetime.

If you're not good at problem management, you may tend to be somewhat disorganized, habitually late, or a chronic procrastinator. These problems tend to make stress much worse, because they prolong negative situations, and things never really get resolved. Over time, thinking and worrying about a problem gets in the way of actually solving it.

GOOD MOVE

Getting upset about uncontrollable stressors can create lots of frustration and needless worry. Next time, and every time, you feel yourself getting upset about something, ask yourself if there's anything you can do to improve the situation. If the answer is no, see if you can "let it be."

There are many spiritual and philosophical approaches to letting go of anger, fear, and sadness that arise in response to the things we can't control. Many of them involve putting the issue into a larger context and accepting the fact that things are the way they are, and we can control only our responses to them.

Healthy Coping

Healthy strategies for emotional regulation allow you to feel what you're feeling, accept it, and find constructive ways to soothe yourself. Emotional regulation isn't about avoiding emotion—it's about healthy expression of emotion and release of tension. Here are some examples of good emotional regulation:

- Talking with a close friend about how you're feeling

- Taking a brisk walk or getting a good workout

- Journaling about the situation and your feelings

- Practicing a musical instrument or artistic pursuit

- Yoga, stretching, and other relaxing exercises

- Listening to music you enjoy

Problem management is all about making things better. Obviously, this type of coping is only appropriate in the face of stressors you have some control over. Also, problem management is most effective if you start with emotional regulation—that is, getting calm and focused before taking action. Here are some good problem-management strategies:

- Making lists, budgets, and schedules

- Enlisting help from friends

- Breaking big problems down into smaller, more manageable steps

- Seeking help from a professional to take care of the problem

Identifying Your Stress Triggers

Everyone gets stressed out sometimes, and each of us has our own unique set of stress triggers. The best way to minimize stress is to catch yourself in the early stages of a stress response. Also, if you know the specific circumstances and situations that cause you stress, you may be able to find ways to avoid them or at least be prepared for them.

Here's a very useful exercise for getting to know your stress buttons better. For one entire day, every time you feel mad, sad, or worried, note it in your journal. Write down exactly what the issue is and what emotion is coming up for you.

GOOD MOVE

Learn to read your body's responses to stressful thoughts—this can give you a head start on coping. Do you clench your jaw or fists, raise your shoulders, get butterflies in your stomach? When you know your body's stress signals, you can be more proactive in preventing full-blown stress attacks.

At the end of the day, or sometime the next day, go over your list. For each item, ask yourself if your negative feelings came about as a result of any of the types of faulty thinking previously described. Then make a note of how you coped with each issue. How many times did you cope with avoidance, eating, or any other unhealthy response? Then, for those stressors that you have some control over, see if you can come up with a healthier, constructive response.

Stress Can Make You Mad, Sad, or Scared

Stressful, threatening appraisals and faulty patterns of thinking lead to negative emotions. The most common emotions associated with stress are anger, fear or worry, and sadness. These are all normal, healthy emotions—but they're uncomfortable. It's very common for people to want to get rid of them as quickly as possible—and this desire leads to quick fixes and avoidant behaviors.

The first step to handling these emotions is to simply let them be. When you deny, suppress, or ignore your feelings, you're not allowing them to come and go naturally. Suppressed emotion has long been recognized as a common cause of anxiety, irritability, and stress-related ailments like fatigue and headache. So next time you're feeling sad, mad, or scared, just let yourself feel that way for a little while. Sometimes it's helpful even to say it out loud: "I'm feeling mad about this right now." In most cases, simply noticing and allowing bad moods to occur leads to their gradual dissipation.

Emotional Stress Leads to Fat

As you've seen, brain levels of feel-good neurotransmitters tend to decline during stressful times. Comfort foods can cause transient elevations in these neurotransmitters. This makes comfort eating seem like a good remedy for stress. Unfortunately, eating junk food in the face of elevated cortisol is the perfect recipe for belly fat.

RED FLAG

A study published by the American Psychological Association in 2007 reported that 43 percent of the 2,000 people surveyed said stress caused them to overeat or eat unhealthy foods. Make sure you're not in that 43 percent!

To lose your belly, you need to find ways to handle bad moods without food or drink. The best way to do this is through exercise, because you get the double benefit of burning calories while not eating junky food that packs the fat on—and the added bonus of the endorphins that are produced during the exercise, which really can help you to feel better. A 15- to 20-minute walk is a wonderful way to release the tension that comes with negative emotion and stress. Another fun option is to turn on some music you like and dance to it for a few minutes. This doesn't solve the problem, but it helps you ride out your emotional response to it so you can deal with it more effectively.

Emotional Balance Leads to Healthier Eating

Over time, as you recognize and accept the thoughts and feelings that come up in response to your daily challenges and stressors, you'll be better able to keep yourself from being overly reactive to them. You will learn that it's possible to feel upset without running away from it or thoughtlessly acting on your emotions. As you become more aware and balanced and tolerant of the shifting sands of your emotional life, you'll find it easier to drop any unhealthy coping behaviors you may have learned in the past. In so doing, you'll also find it easier to lose your belly fat.

The Least You Need to Know

- Stress in your body arises in response to stressful perceptions.
- Coping is what you do whenever you feel overwhelmed or threatened.
- Coping involves managing your emotions and problem solving—and you can replace unhealthy coping strategies with healthy ones.
- Anger, worry, and sadness are the most common emotional responses associated with stress, and they should be acknowledged rather than suppressed.

Three Paths to Being Calmer and Leaner

In This Chapter

- Stress management is essential to belly fat loss
- Meditation generates a quieter mind in a calmer body
- Two types of meditation to try
- Guided imagery and a healthier you

In Chapter 8, we covered a variety of ways to reorganize and reframe your thought processes so you can become less reactive and vulnerable to stressful life events. This is an important first step to good stress management. The next step is to learn some specific skills you can use any time to calm your body and quiet your mind on even your most rushed and busy days.

You release belly fat faster and easier if you spend some time each day training your body and mind to withstand the hassles and challenges of life without undue shocks to your system.

The three techniques described in this chapter—the relaxation response, mindfulness meditation, and guided imagery—are mainstays of mind-body medicine. They've been tested in extensive research, and they've been proven to lower cortisol levels and blood pressure. People who practice one or more of these techniques regularly have been found to have fewer bad moods, less anxiety and worry, and fewer stress-related symptoms such as headaches, fatigue, and insomnia. There are also studies linking the drop in cortisol with successful weight loss.

Give all three types of mind-body stress management a try, then choose the one that appeals to you most (or all of them!) and make a commitment to practicing for 15 to 20 minutes every day. The effects of stress management are cumulative—that is, every bit you do will help.

Meditation

Meditation is a way of quieting your mind and allowing your body to relax in that quiet. It's been a part of every known spiritual and religious tradition throughout history, but it doesn't have to be part of a spiritual practice. Quite simply, learning to meditate means learning to relax into a state in which your mind is quiet and peaceful but still focused, and your body is profoundly relaxed.

Meditation is defined as the intentional self-regulation of attention. It involves settling your focus on one simple thing while allowing your thoughts to drift lazily into and out of your field of attention. People who meditate regularly gain tremendous benefits from it, and feeling calmer and less reactive to everyday stressors is only the beginning.

GOOD MOVE

A regular meditation practice has been demonstrated to increase the production of serotonin in the brain. Serotonin is a neurotransmitter that affects mood and behavior. Low levels of serotonin have been associated with depression, insomnia, headaches, and obesity.

The goal of meditation, no matter what type you're doing, is to bring your full awareness, with all your senses but without judgment, into the present moment and simply "be."

Meditation is helpful because it's all about being quiet, staying calm, and letting thoughts flow by without reacting to them. It's a way to get to know yourself better and to give yourself a break from the constant rush of daily life.

Recent research has found two other very exciting benefits gained by people who meditate regularly that explain why meditators tend to age more slowly than nonmeditators. For one, it's been shown that they experience a reduction in the thinning of the cerebral cortex that occurs with aging. The cerebral cortex is the part of your brain that thinks, perceives, and plans. Degeneration of this area is what leads to the dementia of old age and Alzheimer's disease. In addition, meditation is associated with the optimal function of more than 2,200 *genes* that code for all types of enzymes, including some that protect the body against oxidative damage and regulate energy production.

DEFINITION

A **gene** holds the basic information to build and maintain an organism, as well as pass hereditary information to offspring. Various genes correspond to various traits such as eye color, certain diseases, and areas where we tend to gain weight.

There has been some interesting research on the use of meditation for weight loss, and interesting studies are being conducted at Duke University and other prestigious medical centers. In one group of studies, a type of meditation similar to mindfulness was used successfully to help people be more aware of their bodies' cues about hunger and satiety. Participants in this research have reported significant changes in their eating habits (eating less food at meals and less snacking) within days of beginning to practice. Meditation has also been shown to dramatically reduce bingeing behaviors in both men and women.

There are two types of meditation used most often in stress management and preventative medicine research: the relaxation response and mindfulness-based stress management. Both types involve taking a few minutes every day to sit quietly with yourself and both have been proven to be powerful stress busters.

The Relaxation Response

The relaxation response (RR) is a form of meditation originally developed by Dr. Herbert Benson at Boston's Beth Israel Hospital in the late 1970s. The RR is similar to the ancient practice of transcendental meditation (TM), which originated in India hundreds of years ago. While the term "relaxation response" actually refers to the physiological state of relaxation which results from the quiet focusing of the mind, it's often used to refer to a specific type of mantra-based meditation.

Benson and his colleagues observed remarkable changes in the bodily functions of people while they were engaged in RR, including significant reductions in heart rate and blood pressure, and a shift in brain wave activity to a relaxed *alpha-wave pattern*. These changes are exactly counter to the state you're in when you're chronically or acutely stressed. Since this early research, literally hundreds of papers documenting the positive health benefits of the RR have been published.

DEFINITION

Alpha-wave patterns are typically between 8 to 12 Hz and are generated in a synchronized pattern between the left and right hemispheres of the brain. They are experienced when the mind and body are in a state of complete relaxation and happen more often when the eyes are closed. Some of the benefits of increasing alpha brain waves include increased creativity, a boosted immune system, improved learning ability, balanced mood, and an ability to perform at peak levels.

The RR produces a pleasant, relaxed state of body and mind when you're doing it, but that's not all there is to it. During a meditation session, the body's consumption of oxygen drops to levels below those that occur during sleep. What this amounts to is a few minutes of profound rest for your body at the cellular level. When oxygen consumption goes down for a little while, all the cells of your body get a break from metabolizing sugar and oxygen to make energy—a process that, as you've seen, can load up cells with toxic oxygen-free radicals. So the RR is basically a nonfood antioxidant!

The practice is simple. All you need is about 15 to 20 minutes of uninterrupted quiet time. Find a comfortable spot to sit down. You might be more comfortable if you take off your shoes and glasses (if you wear them), and loosen any tight clothing.

Start by getting comfortable, then closing your eyes and paying attention to your breath. All relaxation exercises start with this—the quiet observation of your breath flowing into and out of your body. It can be even more soothing to breathe in through your nose and out through your mouth while consciously letting go of your body's tension and your mind's concerns.

Next, think about drawing in your breath all the way into your abdomen. For about 3 to 5 minutes, just relax and think about letting each breath flow a little more slowly and a little more deeply into your torso. Now it's time to focus on your mantra.

You have complete freedom to choose any short phrase you'd like for your mantra. Ideally, it's something simple and positive. Some examples include "Let … Go" or "Easy … Breathing" or "Quiet … Mind … Easy … Body." Say the first word silently to yourself as you inhale slowly. Say the second silently on each exhale. This is a great way to keep your attention firmly focused on your breath. It also gives you a "handle" to rely on when your busy mind tries to intrude with all kinds of thoughts—and it will!

Continue sitting quietly, pairing your mantra with your breath, for ten more minutes. At first, it may be hard to avoid getting caught up in the activity of your normally active brain, but over time, you'll notice that you can stay still and calm longer and longer, allowing thoughts to simply glide past.

Mindfulness Meditation

Mindfulness meditation is a practice that's been studied and promoted by John Kabat-Zin at Harvard University for the past 25 years. Mindfulness meditation differs from the relaxation response in that instead of focusing on a word or phrase to keep your attention centered, you simply try to stay fully present to each passing moment.

WHAT'S NEW

A recent study on Mindful Eating and Living (MEAL) demonstrated that using the practice of mindful meditation to reprogram attitudes around food for 6 weeks not only provided the participants with statistically significant weight loss, they also experienced decreases in depression, binge eating, and stress, and an increase in cardiovascular health.

Mindfulness-based stress management is the application of mindfulness meditation to a lifestyle program that's centered around being as aware and present in each moment as one can be. Mindfulness is an attitude or orientation to life that promotes the nonjudgmental participation in your moment to moment existence. There are many ways to apply the attitude of mindfulness to your daily life.

For example, Chapter 10 discusses mindful eating. You can learn to bring this mindful attitude to just about anything you do, from taking a shower to washing the dishes after dinner, to making love. Kabat-Zin and his colleagues at Harvard have studied mindfulness-based stress management for 20 years and they have had great success in relieving the symptoms and progression of a wide range of health problems including high blood pressure, migraine headaches, asthma, and psoriasis.

To practice mindfulness meditation, you begin the same way as with the relaxation response. Find a block of time from 15 to 20 minutes long. Make sure you won't be disturbed and that you are in a comfortable place. Get comfortable, loosen any tight clothing, take off your shoes, and sit quietly for a few moments. The next step is to close your eyes and direct your attention to your breath. Without trying to change anything, simply notice your breath entering through your nose and filling your chest, and slowly leaving through your mouth. Continue sitting quietly and observing your breathing for a few minutes.

In mindfulness meditation, the goal is to simply sit quietly and notice what is going on around you and inside you. In addition, the goal is to avoid attaching a positive or negative value or judgment to your experience. This type of meditation is one that challenges you to observe your flow of thoughts without being distracted or stimulated by them. Mindfulness meditation is especially helpful for stress management because as you practice, you become aware that many of your thoughts are simply chatter generated by habit. When you're meditating like this, you begin to create a brief moment between thinking a thought and having an emotional reaction to it.

GOOD MOVE

It's not uncommon to feel frustrated by distractions when you are trying to meditate. Distractions are normal and it is the work of mindfulness meditation to learn to accept and deal with your brain chatter. When a distraction arises, simply observe the distraction, release it without judgment, and return your focus to your breathing.

Over time, as you practice mindfulness meditation, you'll become more and more aware of that little space between having a thought and reacting to it emotionally. People who meditate regularly have been found to be happier, calmer, and more resilient to stress. You'll find it a natural inclination to bring a mindful, relaxed attitude to many of the things you do all day long.

Guided Imagery

Guided imagery is an activity that involves deliberately generating images in your mind while in a relaxed state. Guided imagery has been used for many years by many people coping with stress illness and anxiety. Guided imagery has also been used extensively in the world of sports and theater to enhance performance. And more recently guided imagery has been used as an adjunct to diet and exercise in many weight-loss programs.

When you use guided imagery, you are communicating with your body in the most direct way possible. Imagery is nonverbal, sensory information, and this is how the body and mind communicate best with each other. If you think about something happening, for example an argument or other stressful situation, the more vividly you imagine and remember it, the more likely you are to feel the physical side of that event. For many people, these little "mind movies" run spontaneously and repeatedly all day long. And every time the movie plays, it generates anywhere between a mild level of activation to a full-blown fight or flight state.

GOOD MOVE

Even 10 minutes of guided imagery meditation have been shown to reduce blood pressure, lower cholesterol, reduce pain, and even reduce blood loss during surgery, resulting in better surgical outcomes. For this reason, insurance companies have begun to provide patients with guided imagery CDs pre-operation.

So you see, you are using imagery all the time. Every time you think about something that happened in the past or that might happen in the future, your body reacts as if it were really happening, at least to some extent. The more time you spend thinking about bad, scary, or sad things, the more frequently throughout your day your body will be activated into a stress state. And as you've seen, many of us cope with that activation by reaching for something tasty to eat. Guided imagery is helpful for stress because it gets you into the habit of imagining positive and pleasant experiences regularly.

There are some important things to remember when you start using guided imagery. First of all, imagery is not visualization—it's so much more. The most effective guided imagery exercises involve all of your senses. Daydreams, memories, and other types of mental imagery are more immediate and vivid when they include sounds, textures, smells, and even tastes.

Another requirement for the best use of guided imagery is to be relaxed, calm, and focused when you practice. When you put your mind and body into a relaxed state, your entire system becomes more receptive to the thoughts and images you generate. Finally, research in the use of guided imagery for health care has demonstrated that soothing, pleasant music also seems to enhance the effectiveness of the imagery exercise.

See It and Make It Real

In the world of sports, imagery has been used extensively to enhance performance. In the world of medicine, imagery has been used to produce a wide variety of physical phenomena and better health. All of these functions of imagery come about because the body responds to the mind's images by becoming more like what's being imagined. It's almost as if vivid imagery produces a sort of template or model that the body does its best to follow.

Athletes are trained to use imagery to improve concentration and to reduce performance anxiety. Also, they're taught to rehearse their skills using vivid, multisensory imagery. In this method, a specific action, such as serving a tennis ball, is imagined happening in slow motion while the athlete vividly evokes all the complex muscular and sensory components of the activity. Doing this type of rehearsal over and over again has been shown to dramatically improve performance.

GOOD MOVE

Meditation has been proven to provide the mind with an increased level of creativity and performance. Check out this list of famous people who have made meditation part of their daily lives: David Lynch (film maker), Russell Simmons (music producer), Apolo Ohno (speed skater), Jim Carrey (film star and comedian), and Jet Li (martial arts star).

In medicine, guided imagery has produced a wide variety of measurable, significant physical states that enhance health and healing. People scheduled for surgery who practice guided imagery before the procedure tend to be less anxious pre-operatively, lose less blood and require less anesthesia during the operation, and are released from the hospital more quickly and with fewer complications than those who don't.

You can use imagery in your belly fat loss program in both of the ways described—for stress reduction and for building confidence and motivation like an athlete. The following exercise is designed to help you relax and create a vision of the healthy body you can achieve by losing belly fat with this program.

A Sample Guided Imagery Exercise

What follows is a short guided imagery script. I recommend that you ask a friend or family member to read it to you the first time you try it. Better yet, make a recording of yourself reading it aloud. Use the recording for your daily practice. If you decide to record the script, make sure you speak slowly, with a calm, soothing voice. Another alternative is to ask someone you love to record it for you.

When you do guided imagery, it's helpful to have soothing, peaceful music that you enjoy playing during the exercise. To start, sit down in a comfortable place where you won't be disturbed for several minutes. Make sure you aren't distracted by uncomfortable clothing. Set the intention to communicate with your body in a caring, positive way, and then begin:

GOOD MOVE

Here is a list of great musical CDs to get you started with guided imagery:

- *Slow World* by Liquid Mind (1996) Real Music/Chuck Wild Records
- *Angel Love* by Aeoliah (1998) Oreade Music
- *Earth Spirit* by R. Carlos Nakai (1993) Canyon Records
- *Inner Peace* by Steven Halpern (2002) Inner Peace Music

Relax into your seat and let go of any tension you can feel in your jaw and your neck. Imagine the muscles becoming softer and looser with every breath you take. Now see this relaxation spreading to your shoulders, down both your arms, and to your hands. As you focus on releasing the tension in your upper body, allow your breath to move gently and freely, in through your nose and out through your mouth. A nice way to consciously relax the muscles of your arms and legs is to imagine they are becoming comfortably warm and heavy.

Allow your chest and belly to gently expand a tiny bit more with each breath that comes in. Imagine all of your muscles relaxing just a bit more with each breath you exhale. Continue in this way, focusing on expansion as you inhale, and release as you exhale. With each breath, your body will naturally let go of stress and move into a calmer, healthier state.

For the next two or three minutes, continue your calm, gentle observation of your breath as it flows in through your nose and out through your mouth. If distracting thoughts intrude, simply notice them and let them fade as you consistently return your attention to your breath.

Now, imagine that you are in a beautiful, healthy, safe place. This can be a real place you've visited before or someplace you've imagined. The most important thing is that you feel comfortable and safe in this place. Take a look around at all there is to see in this lovely safe place, noticing light and color and movement and anything else that catches your eye.

Pay attention to the sounds you can hear in this safe place. As you move around, you may also notice pleasant smells and textures. Keep in mind that this is your own safe place, so you can remove anything that doesn't please and comfort you. Also, you can bring in anything that you think would make this place more delightful and comfortable for you.

Now, imagine that you have lost all the weight and belly fat you need to lose. Imagine that you have learned to eat and exercise and manage stress so well that your body is lean and strong and full of calm energy. Imagine that you can look into a mirror and see yourself and your body the way you want to be.

As you experience this thinner, healthier you, don't just focus on what you look like. Pay attention to how your body feels now that you've gotten rid of the weight you didn't need. What are you wearing? What emotions are coming up for you? What's your energy level? Notice what it's like to breathe and walk and simply be in your body now that it's healthier and leaner.

As you appreciate and really feel what it's like to have the body you want, remind yourself that you can make this happen. In fact, just by doing this exercise, you're moving another step closer to your goal. Remember that you have everything you need to eat well, get regular exercise, and manage stress every day.

Take another moment to imagine yourself at your goal weight, feeling confident, strong, and happy. And now, knowing that you can return to your safe place any time you want or need to, return your attention to your breathing.

Feel your breath entering and leaving your body, and then slowly start to move your fingers and toes, bringing your awareness fully into the here and now. Take one last slow deep breath, and open your eyes.

Many people find it useful to record any thoughts and feelings that come up while doing this and other meditative exercises. You might want to keep your journal handy to jot down any new ideas or observations that come to you.

Yoga for a Serene Mind and Supple Body

Yoga has become an immensely popular way of staying relaxed and flexible, and keeping slim. The word yoga means "union" in Sanskrit, referring to the union of mind, body, and spirit that results from practice. We can also think of yoga as a way to unite mind, breath, and body.

It seems that any practice that gets your breath and body movements in sync has a powerful effect on the nervous system, inducing deep relaxation and focus. Examples of this include mindful walking, Tai Chi, Chi Gong, and, of course, yoga. Yoga is a great form of active meditation, leaving you feeling calm but also energized when you're done.

Health Benefits of Yoga

Yoga has been studied extensively as a way to relax, and also as a method of rehabilitation and illness management. The bodily benefits of yoga include more supple joints, less muscle stiffness and back pain, and fewer headaches. Beyond that, yoga offers many psychological and emotional benefits.

Yoga has been shown to produce a drop in blood levels of epinephrine, cortisol, and blood pressure after each session. It can also help lower levels of norepinephrine in the brain, which makes you feel calmer and happier. Yoga has also been shown to increase brain levels of oxytocin, the "trust and bonding" hormone, which helps you feel more relaxed and connected to other people.

Yoga at Home—A Simple Stretch

You don't need any equipment or special clothing to bring this simple yoga routine into your everyday life. I recommend doing this routine first thing in the morning and right before bed to keep your muscles well-nourished and relaxed.

Step 1: Standing toward the front of your mat, place your feet hip-width apart. Stand up tall with your arms relaxed by your sides. Inhale; reach your arms up toward the ceiling. As you exhale, bring your hands to the prayer position in front of your chest.

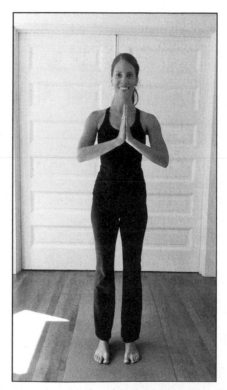

Standing tall with your shoulders relaxed, knees loose, and hands in the prayer position.

Inhale; straighten and lengthen your spine up from your lower back through the crown of your head. As you exhale, hinge at your hips and fold forward, reaching for your toes.

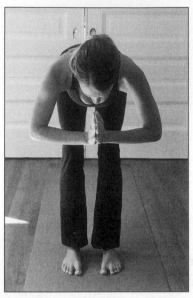

Bending forward with feet planted firmly on the mat.

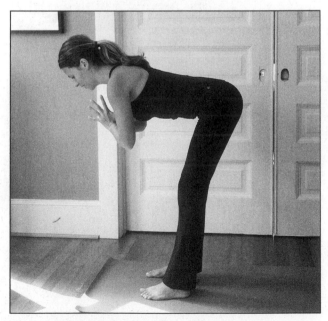

Keep your back straight and your knees loose. They can bend as much as needed to avoid straining your lower back.

Step 2: Bend your knees and plant your palms on the floor. Take care not to strain your lower back—bend your knees if you need to in order to touch the floor. Keeping your hands where they are, take a few steps back with your feet until your hips are bent at about a 45 degree angle and your buttocks are sticking straight up in the air, with your back straight. Your body should look like an upside down V. Gently press your heels down toward the floor. This is downward facing dog.

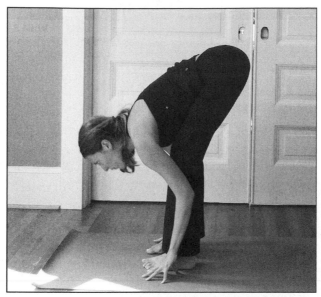

With your hands touching the floor, extend your neck to look straight down at your mat.

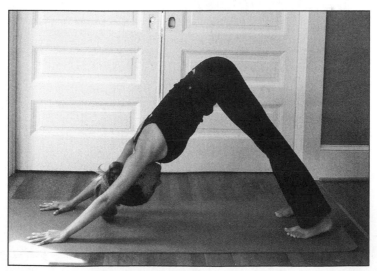

Downward dog is an excellent hamstring stretch. Lift your heels as much as you need to.

Step 3: Hold the downward facing dog position for another 3 breaths, focusing on getting full expansion of your chest with each inhale and releasing tension in the back of your legs and lower back with each exhale.

Take another deep breath in, and as you exhale, bend your knees, lowering them all the way to your yoga mat. This is tabletop.

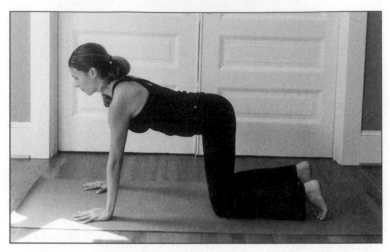

On all fours, make sure your shoulders and hips are directly over your hands and knees.

Step 4: Untuck your toes and drop your hips back to your heels, placing your forehead on the floor. Your arms should be lying relaxed on the floor, parallel to your torso. This is child's pose.

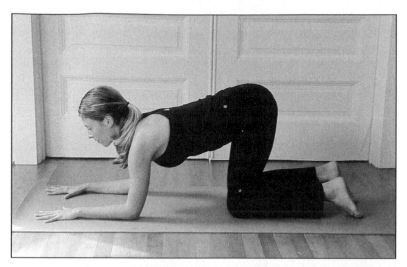

Stay loose and relaxed, and if you feel any strain, ease out of the position.

Stay here for another three or four slow, deep breaths, or as long as 5 minutes or so, feeling your entire spine relax into this gentle stretch.

Step 5: When you're ready, take another slow breath in and as you do, lift your body back up to tabletop, standing on all fours with your shoulders stacked over your wrists and your hips over your knees.

Step 6: Tuck your toes under, lift your hips high, and push back into downward facing dog. From this position, walk your feet forward to meet your hands at the front of your yoga mat.

Step 7: Inhale, and then as you exhale, slowly and deliberately straighten your spine one vertebrae at a time, until you're standing up straight with your arms hanging relaxed at your sides. Take another deep breath in, and release it in a long, slow exhale.

Repeat this sequence at least once, ideally up to 4 times, to get the full benefit of the stretches and the invigorating movements. Practice this routine on most mornings, and over time you'll notice that your back and legs feel looser, more relaxed, and less stiff. You'll be training yourself to pay more attention to your body's signals and what it needs as your belly shrinks.

The Least You Need to Know

- Practicing a stress management technique for 15 minutes a day will reduce cortisol levels and sympathetic nervous system activity, accelerating your belly fat loss.

- Meditation is a process of quieting and focusing your mind, leading to better moods and reduction of stress physiology as well as slower aging.

- Guided imagery is a technique for "seeing" yourself more relaxed and thinner and has been proven to induce real changes in behavior, performance, and physical health.

Eating Away at Belly Fat

Wherever you go food surrounds you—at the gas station, convenience store, department store, and practically on every corner. With so much food readily available it's easy to eat without thinking and without really being hungry. People also eat in a hurry, on the road, and while doing other things—and even worse, late at night. On the other hand, you often miss the most important meal of the day—breakfast. All of these things contribute to belly fat. This part will teach you how to turn your diet upside down and eat when you're hungry—becoming a more mindful eater—eat in the morning and throughout the day, and stop eating at night. In return you'll have more energy, be able to think clearer, be in a better mood, improve sleep patterns, and be able to digest your food better.

Mindless Eating

In This Chapter

- How mindless eating impacts belly fat
- What it means to eat mindlessly
- What the benefits are of mindful eating
- How to make a change in your habits

Have you ever plowed your way through a huge plate of spaghetti and sat back feeling stuffed, uncomfortable, and unable to remember a single bite? If so, you've experienced the trap of mindless eating.

Mindless eating is a common way that many people pile on belly fat. This is because when you eat mindlessly, you can consume hundreds of calories above and beyond what you need at that moment and not enjoy a single one. This happens when you aren't noticing how the food is making you feel when you eat it, so you miss all your body's signals that it's had enough—time to put down your fork (or that bag of chips)! Also, mindless eating usually means eating things that aren't good for you.

In his book *Mindless Eating*, leading food-behavior researcher, Brian Wansink, explains that our environment and our social conditioning encourage us to eat mindlessly. It's a part of modern American life to eat out of habit or according to a schedule, or even the social expectations of other people—all reasons that have little or nothing to do with hunger and what our bodies actually need.

Here we discuss what it means to be a mindless eater, why it's bad for your belly, and how you can become a mindful eater. Mindful eating does more than just control your weight and slim down your middle, it also increases your enjoyment of food so that every meal (or at least most of them) can be a good one.

Eating While Distracted or Multitasking

Many people have a hard time sitting down to eat without some type of distraction, especially when eating alone. This is a problem because it keeps you from being aware of how your body is reacting to the food—so you don't get the full enjoyment available from the act of eating, and you don't know when to stop eating. Whether you've pulled into a drive-thru while rushing through your errands, or worked at your computer while absentmindedly taking bite after bite, it's easy to feel that there's no time to stop and focus on eating.

A simple test of your reliance on distraction is to see how you feel about sitting down alone with a plate of food with nothing else to look at. Do you feel resistant to doing that? Read on—you'll find many reasons to try it—and you'll start enjoying your snacks and meals all the more.

If you often eat at home by yourself, it's very easy to fall into the habit of eating every meal and snack while watching television or cruising the internet. In the battle for your attention, chances are the screen usually wins, and you miss out on the experience of eating—and the stop signals that keep you from overeating. To break this habit, start with one meal a day.

Set the table as you would if you had a guest joining you. Choose a seat with a nice view out a window, if possible. Put your condiments on the table and pour yourself a glass of water. Now, put on some enjoyable, soothing music. This will help you relax and focus on eating. The music and the scenery will provide some entertainment, but not enough to completely distract you from your food.

GOOD MOVE

When it comes to changing eating habits and thinking mindfully, many people feel overwhelmed. To make things easy, try thinking in terms of three. Decide on three changes you can do mindlessly and without much sacrifice, such as turning off the TV or just taking one portion. Then just do it. Small changes mean a lot.

Eating in a Hurry

If you eat while running around getting things done, you're eating in a highly activated state—a state in which you simply cannot digest and absorb your food at optimal levels.

It's very easy to find things to eat while on the run—convenience foods are everywhere, from the gas station to the hardware store. Sadly, these foods are almost universally over-processed and laden with unhealthy fats, sugars, and too much salt—exactly the types of foods most strongly linked with belly fat. Add in the sugared drinks in the vending machines you see everywhere you go, and you have a surefire recipe for a bloated belly.

WHAT'S NEW

It's estimated that 80 percent of all car accidents are caused by distracted drivers. While cell phone use and texting get the most attention, a significant number of these crashes happen because the drivers are distracted by eating and drinking while driving. The worst offenders are hamburgers and coffee.

It's not just quality that counts—it's quantity. When you grab and eat without paying attention, it's so easy to eat more than what you need without really appreciating any of it. Portion sizes in convenience foods have more than doubled in the last 20 years, so eating a bag of chips nowadays may mean consuming up to 3 servings! Beverages, too, have ballooned; nearly all bottled drinks, such as ice tea, contain two servings.

Eating Food Because It's There

Many people are in the habit of eating simply because food is present. There's a bowl of popcorn in the room—everyone starts munching and they don't stop until the bowl is empty. If you ask them why, they usually don't have an answer! Because it was there? This isn't a good way to manage your nutritional needs. The point isn't to sit there and deprive yourself, but to pay attention! Decide how much you're going to eat, take that much, and enjoy eating it. Then notice that you aren't hungry any more (ideally you didn't eat any at all unless you were hungry to begin with), and shift your focus to something else.

Sometimes, when there isn't anything else to do, people eat just to entertain themselves or to pass the time. In airports, the terminals abound with all kinds of fast food stops and they're usually full of people eating and drinking. Chances are, most of these people are eating simply because there's very little else to do at the airport. More and more, it seems that food is offered as a way to keep us entertained rather than nourished.

The "Clean Your Plate" Syndrome

Many of us grew up being told to eat everything on our plates at mealtime. There seemed to be a moral obligation to children elsewhere in the world to clean our plates—as if that would somehow end world hunger. While parents who insist on the "leave no crumb behind" policy may mean well, it's long been thought that they may be inadvertently setting their children up for being overweight or obese. Several studies of the eating behavior of children have found that this may very well be true. Kids younger than three or four tend to stop eating when they're full, whether or not their plates are clean. After the age of four or so, however, a child's food intake is heavily influenced by portion sizes—the bigger the plate of food, the more they'll eat.

Kids aren't the only ones who eat until the food is gone. Adults are also avid plate cleaners, and this behavior doesn't appear to be strongly linked to parental demands during childhood. Instead, adults seem to be conditioned to keep eating until the food is gone. The reasons for this may include eating "when it's time to eat" instead of when you're hungry, and the tendency to keep eating as long as your dining partner continues to eat.

RED FLAG

If you have oversized plates in your kitchen cupboard, you could be eating more than you need without even noticing it. Research shows people given 12-inch plates ate an average 22 percent more food than people given 10-inch plates in a laboratory eating study—and when asked at the end of the experiment, they weren't aware that they had eaten more. So get yourself a set of smaller plates and you'll be eating less without even noticing it!

The Mindless Eating Questionnaire

Let's take a minute and find out if mindless eating is an issue for you. Take this simple quiz to increase your understanding of your own tendencies for mindless, automatic eating behavior. Rate each item on the quiz based on how often it occurs in your life—ranging from "rarely" to "several times a day." When you're done, add up your score.

The Mindless Eating Questionnaire

Rate each item based on how often you do each of these behaviors in your regular routine using this scale:

Never or almost never: 1
Once or twice a week: 2
Every day: 3
Several times a day: 4

How often do you ...   **Response**

1. Eat while watching television   _____

2. Take something to read when you're dining out alone _____

3. Eat while driving your car   _____

4. Eat food just because it's there   _____

5. Eat while sitting at your desk   _____

6. Finish a meal only when your plate is empty   _____

7. Eat while reading a book or magazine   _____

8. Start picking up your next bite before you're finished chewing the food in your mouth   _____

9. Eat because you saw someone on television eating   _____

10. Eat while talking on the phone   _____

11. Finish a snack or meal with little or no memory of each bite you took   _____

12. Eat while walking down the street   _____

13. Finish a snack or meal and feel surprised at how much you ate   _____

14. Eat while standing up in the kitchen   _____

Your overall score is an indication of your general tendency to eat without paying attention. While most of us do some of these things every now and then, it's a problem when this type of eating becomes a daily habit.

If your score is between 14 and 30, you probably have a moderate tendency to distract yourself while you eat, and you'll make better progress toward your flat belly by practicing the mindful eating tips in this chapter.

If your score is over 30, you may find that making the shift to mindful eating is a big change—and making it will be a huge boost toward your goal of losing belly fat. Be patient with yourself and consider this a chance to explore.

The "French Paradox"

The "French Paradox" is the term used by many to describe the phenomenon of low obesity rates in France (compared to those in the United States) in spite of a standard diet rich in meat, cheese, and simple carbohydrates.

The traditional French approach to eating involves slowing down and enjoying food, and allowing all kinds of food to be part of a healthy, balanced lifestyle. A study done at Cornell University found that people from the United States, compared to people from France, are much more likely to stop eating based on external cues rather than internal ones such as feeling full or satisfied.

Americans reported that they stop eating when they've eaten an amount of food that other people would consider "normal," when it's getting late, when their TV show ends, or when they finish what they're reading. The French subjects in the study were much less likely to be swayed by these types of cues—instead, they reported that they stopped eating when they felt satisfied or no longer hungry—the result of the body's natural responses to taking in food.

GOOD MOVE

One easy way to reduce mindless eating at mealtimes is to avoid serving food "family style," with heaping platters on the table. While interacting with your family and friends, it's easy to take two or even three servings of food that you aren't even hungry for without noticing. Leave the food in the kitchen and prepare a plate to take to the table with you. Then, taking seconds becomes a conscious choice.

One approach to avoiding eating mindlessly is to adopt some features of the traditional French style of eating: make every meal an event to be enjoyed; allow yourself to eat food you like in moderation without stressing about it; balance a big meal with one or two smaller meals that day; eat slowly, and stop when you're satisfied—and you'll know when you're satisfied because you're eating slowly and paying attention to how your body feels!

Sadly, obesity rates in France are beginning to climb at an alarming rate, and this trend has been attributed to a slow shift away from their traditional way of eating and toward a more rushed, stressful style that's now typical in the United States.

The Solution: Mindful Eating

We're creatures of habit, and habit is an economical way to behave—you don't have to think about everything you do because a lot of it is automatic. You don't have to remember how to drive every time you start up your car, for example, or think carefully about the route to work. You just get going and soon, you're there. Being mindful doesn't mean being obsessive about every little detail of your daily routine, but it does involve paying more attention to what you're doing and how you feel while you're doing it.

Mindful eating is paying attention to food and the act of eating. It's also the practice of noticing how your body and mind respond to the different foods you eat. A key component of mindful eating is to notice these things without automatically labeling them as good or bad. A mindful eater eats when she's hungry, and eats only the amount of food required to stop feeling hungry. This simple shift in eating behavior can go a long way toward getting rid of belly fat.

You'll Eat Less

Research has shown over and over again that mindful eaters consistently eat less at each meal and fewer snacks than mindless eaters do. In addition, their recall of what they ate is more accurate. There are two basic ways this works. First, mindful eaters are better at predicting how much food they're going to need to eat to satisfy their hunger. They allow that feeling to guide them in how much food they serve themselves—so their plates begin less full than one that was mindlessly piled up.

Secondly, becoming a mindful eater means learning how your stomach feels when it's beginning to get full and you've had enough to eat. At first, these signals may seem subtle and easy to miss, but with practice, you can easily know when it's time to stop eating.

You'll Make Better Choices

Over time, a mindful eater pays attention to how different foods make him feel. A heavy load of carbs makes him drowsy. A very salty meal leaves him feeling bloated. When you know how your food choices will affect you in the hour or two after you eat them, you can make informed decisions about what and how much to eat.

Interestingly, this type of awareness can enhance your appreciation for healthy foods. It's a simple matter of cause and effect. If eating a healthy breakfast causes you to feel alert and energetic all morning, you'll probably want to eat that breakfast again to reap the same reward.

How to Become a Mindful Eater

Basically, mindful eating is paying attention to your food and your body so you can enjoy the basic act of eating and the delightful essence of food—without being overly critical. Therapists have been using the principle of mindfulness to treat eating disorders for years—and it's been found to be quite helpful for people who overeat.

There's also growing evidence that mindful eating can be helpful to pretty much everyone—especially those of us who live fast-paced, overextended lives. According to the Center for Mindful Eating, eating mindfully involves four things:

- Cultivating a positive attitude toward preparing and eating food
- Using all your senses to savor your food
- Liking or disliking different foods without being overly self-critical
- Learning to follow internal cues to decide when to start and stop eating

Let's take a look at each of these ideas in a little more detail.

Enjoy Cooking and Eating Food

Many of us are resistant to spending a lot of time cooking. If you absolutely refuse to become a cook, you can at least devote some time and research to learning about healthy food. You can prepare it with the intention of nourishing yourself. What this really means is that you need to get involved in feeding yourself! Make smart decisions about what you eat and enjoy your selections.

Furthermore, getting good skills in the kitchen is empowering and helps you feel more in control of the food you cook and eat. Studies show kids who are involved in food production are more likely to eat the healthy food they prepare than if they're not involved. The same holds true for adults.

Appreciate Food with All Five Senses

Eating is a basic human activity that can bring great joy and satisfaction to your life. There's more to food than the taste—it can be beautiful to look at, interesting to feel in your mouth, smell divine, and be fun to pick up and play with. You were given the gift of five senses, and it's a basic tenet of mindfulness that the more of this you bring to every life experience, the more rich and pleasurable it will be.

Take more time to experience the five senses of eating at every meal. Most people eat with their eyes before they even taste the food—why not add touch, smell, and sound to that as well.

Learn What You Like and Don't Like

You don't like broccoli? Okay, that's fine! You can find lots of other highly nutritious vegetables to enjoy. You love sour cream? Great! Find ways to bring a low-fat version of it into your diet in reasonable amounts. The point is to practice nonjudgment when choosing food. Choose food based on whether or not you like it—but make that distinction based on your five-sense conscious eating behavior.

Listen to Your Body

People decide to start eating for all kinds of reasons, and physical hunger frequently isn't one of them. Emotional hunger and sensory hunger are two common triggers for eating. It's important to be able to identify what type of hunger you're feeling when you have an urge to eat. You'll be much more successful at losing your belly fat if you only eat when your body is hungry.

Physical hunger tends to build gradually in the three or four hours after your last meal. Physical hunger makes itself felt in your body, with a hollow feeling in your abdomen and a slight drop in your energy level. Eating a moderate amount of food makes it go away.

All types of hunger begin in your brain, but only physical hunger arises because your body needs fuel. Physical hunger starts in the hypothalamus of your brain, an important structure that is constantly monitoring basic life support information from your body, such as your blood pressure, blood sugar, body temperature, and more. It processes this information without any conscious thought from you and coordinates changes to keep things in balance. Many of these changes are automatic, but some require you to take conscious action, so the hypothalamus can send subtle signals to your higher thinking brain that motivate you to do things such as eating, drinking, or even taking a nap.

As your stomach becomes emptied of the food you ate in your last meal and your blood sugar levels slowly fall, your brain translates that information into your experience of being hungry. It's a beautifully balanced system when it isn't derailed by other types of hunger and mindless eating.

Emotional hunger and sensory hunger also arise in the brain, but not in response to your body's need for food. Emotional hunger tends to arise suddenly, in the midst of feeling sad or anxious, regardless of when you last ate. It tends to be sensed mostly in your mind with no reliable cues from your belly or your energy level. Emotional hunger also doesn't tend to fade easily after eating a moderate amount of food—which is why so many emotional eaters tend to be overeaters.

Sensory hunger is that feeling of desire for a food after smelling, seeing, or tasting it. It's that sudden desire for french fries when you walk past a fast food restaurant or cake at a birthday party. As with emotional hunger, it can arise any time after you last ate and doesn't correspond with your energy level.

To lose your belly fat, you need to learn when you're really hungry and when you just feel like eating for emotional or sensory reasons. Then, you need to pay attention to your body's signals that you've had enough and it's time to stop eating.

Your stop eating signal is called *satiation*. You can only really "hear" this signal if you eat deliberately and without great haste. Slow down. Check in to your body while you're eating. Your stomach, pancreas, and other organs will be secreting an elaborate set of hormones and other chemicals in response to the food you're eating. This takes a few minutes. You need to give your system a chance to send information to your brain about the effects of what you're eating in order to benefit from this primeval wisdom.

DEFINITION

Satiation is the sum of the bodily processes that signal that you've eaten enough. It is the feeling of nonhunger you get after eating. High-calorie, low-quality foods tend to provide minimal satiation and satiety, which may explain why people tend to eat more of them, and feel hungry soon after eating them. So they eat more. Hello, belly fat.

As your stomach distends, it begins stimulating the release of a hormone known as cholecystekinin (CCK). CCK signals your brain that you're getting full and you don't need to eat any more. Your pancreas is churning out insulin in response to the carbohydrates in the food you're eating. If you're healthy, the insulin will travel all over your body and help the process of absorption. One of the things it will do, if you're paying attention, is help you know when you've taken in enough energy and can stop eating for now.

Keep a Food Journal

A food journal or food diary is where you write down everything you eat or drink in a day. People who keep detailed food journals lose more weight and keep that weight off in the long run compared to people who don't keep journals at all. According to one large study tracking nearly 1,700 people, those who kept daily food records lost *twice* as much weight as those who kept no records at all. So what's so special about a food diary?

The simple act of writing down what you eat encourages you to eat less, by increasing your awareness of what, how much, and why you're eating. There are other benefits, too. A food journal helps you identify eating patterns and areas where you can make changes. It can reveal triggers to avoid, such as overeating when out or drinking too much. And, it allows you to compare your eating habits with the ones discussed in this meal plan.

Include the following in your food diary:

- Date
- What you ate
- How much you ate
- When you ate it

- Where you were
- Who you were with
- Exercise you did that day
- Mood you were in

Here are a few tips for successful food journaling:

1. Write down everything you eat, including snacks, candies, tastes, and bites. These can add up quickly. Americans typically underestimate their calorie intake by about 25 percent.

2. Be as detailed and accurate as possible. At first you may need to weigh and measure all of your food, but later on you'll get better at eyeballing amounts. This will give you a better idea of how many calories you're taking in.

3. Write down the food as soon as you finish eating it. If you wait until the end of the day you're likely to forget some things.

4. Review your journal weekly, and then make changes accordingly.

5. Be vigilant—remember the more you write down the more weight you lose.

GOOD MOVE

When it comes to tallying up calorie intake, most people go for the old-fashion pen, paper, and spiral notebook. If you are more high-tech, however, there are many online journals like myfooddiary.com and sparkpeople.com available. These websites actually calculate calories and other nutrients for you. See Appendix B for more sites to check out.

The SAFE Approach to Mindful Eating

Eating food is more than just a habit or a survival skill. It can be a basic pleasure in life. Mindful eating will enhance your health, decrease the amount you eat, and serve as a basic weapon to fight belly fat.

When it's time for a snack or a meal, it's also time to relax and rejuvenate your body. Whatever it is you're going to eat, present it to yourself nicely. This doesn't take much effort, but as you're getting out a small plate and putting the food on it, your brain is busy telling your stomach and the rest of your body that it's about to be fed. Your physiology is going to automatically start shifting into eating mode.

GOOD MOVE

Taking smaller bites and chewing your food thoroughly allows salivary amylase, an enzyme in saliva, to begin the process of digestion. The more slowly you eat, the more effectively this enzyme works to make the nutrients in food more available to your body.

If you also make a conscious decision to slow down a bit and enjoy your food, you'll amplify this effect. You might even find your mouth watering as you get ready to eat, a sure sign that you've given your body time to get ready to eat.

The SAFE technique will help you become a mindful eater. SAFE is an acronym for a ritual you can perform every time you eat—whether it's a snack or a meal. It stands for **S**it down, **A**ttend, **F**irst bite, **E**njoy, and it's an easy to way to remember to make eating mindful and conscious. Whether it's popcorn in a movie theater or a four-course dinner at a fine restaurant, make SAFE eating a habit. It will help you live at a healthy weight, be less stressed, and derive the maximum nutritional benefit from every bite of food you eat. Let's go over each one.

Sit Down

You're not a cow, you're a human being—sit down! As a human being, you're more relaxed when you sit down. It only takes a few minutes to eat a snack, and a little more than that to eat a meal. No matter how busy you are, you probably have time to sit down and focus while you're eating. Make it a rule to eat food only if you're sitting in a chair (not in your car!). When you sit down, your heart rate and blood pressure will slow, and your muscles will naturally relax. Sitting down also sets the intention that you're going to take in this food with deliberation, even if the snack or meal only takes a few minutes.

Attend

Before you eat, look at the food in front of you. Pay attention to the colors, textures, and shapes you can see. Take a minute to inhale the aromas of the food and let that spark your appetite so you're primed and ready when you take that first bite.

First Bite

Focus all your senses on the first bite you take of the food. Take a bite, put down your fork, apple, or whatever you're eating, relax your hands, and savor this first bite. Explore the taste and texture of the food while you're chewing it. Food tells your body it's all right to let down its guard and simply absorb the goodness and bounty that's available. For a little while, at least, all is well and you've got everything you need right in front of you.

Enjoy

Keep eating, paying attention to each bite—perhaps not with the same level of focus as with the first bite, but continue paying attention to how it feels to be eating this food, allowing yourself to enjoy it. When you've eaten half of it, take a break. This is important! Again, put down the food, your fork, or spoon, and check in. Are you still enjoying the food? Are you starting to feel full? Do you need to eat the rest? This is part of learning to follow internal cues, not external ones, to signal having enough. If you develop this as a habit, you'll easily and effortlessly overcome any tendency you may have to overeat. After you've answered these questions, either go ahead and finish the food or call it done and put the rest away for later.

Practice this technique with every snack and meal you eat, and soon you'll find yourself not only eating less, but also enjoying it more. You'll also have the added benefit of knowing your stomach, intestines, pancreas, liver, and all the other players in digestion and absorption are functioning at their best to make the most of every bite.

The Least You Need to Know

- Mindless eating often results in eating more, and choosing less healthy foods.
- Mindless eaters tend to eat while distracted, multitasking, or by force of habit instead of hunger.
- Focusing on the food you're eating increases your enjoyment of it and usually results in eating less.
- Eating because you're hungry and not in response to external cues is a key to healthy eating.

Timing Is Everything

In This Chapter

- The benefits of breakfast
- Small meals stave off hunger
- Family dinners make a difference
- Nighttime eating is a nightmare

In our food centric culture where you can find diners, grocery stores, and fast food restaurants open 24 hours, many people don't think twice about eating any time of the day or night. This constant barrage of food makes it even easier for us to eat or drink something nearly continuously from the time that we wake up to the time that we go to sleep. But, when you eat is just as important as what you eat and in this chapter you see why.

Providing your body with the energy it needs first thing in the morning is crucial to the success of this program and losing weight. It's also particularly important for keeping your tummy trim and slim. Consequently, breakfast plays a huge role in your diet.

Small healthy meals eaten regularly throughout the day are another boon for satisfying hunger without overeating and a good habit to get into, first because we get accustomed to smaller portions and second because it promotes good digestion and boosts metabolism.

Dinner is also one meal you don't want to miss, but it shouldn't be the majority of all your calories either. Eating a light, low-calorie dinner together with your family is the best way to go. And, you should avoid eating late at night—not only will it put on the pounds but it can also disrupt sleep and lead to other unhealthy lifestyles. Read on (but don't stay up too late) to find out more.

The Mechanics of Metabolism

Metabolism refers to the way your body uses energy. Your *basal metabolic rate (BMR)* is the speed at which you burn calories at rest, this includes all your vital functions like breathing, circulating blood, and maintaining body temperature. The majority of your calories, 60 to 75 percent, go to your BMR, another 10 percent is used for the process of digestion and absorption of food, and the rest is for physical activity.

> **DEFINITION**
>
> **Metabolism** is the sum total energy needed for all the chemical reactions that go on in your body.
>
> Your **basal metabolic rate (BMR)** is the rate you burn energy, known as calories, while completely at rest. This includes all of your vital bodily functions.

Metabolic rates vary from individual to individual depending on age, height, genetics, body composition (the more muscle you have the higher your metabolic rate), stress, and a few other things. Physical activity is the most variable of these factors, as the more you exercise the higher your BMR, mainly due to more muscle and less fat. Based on your metabolic rate you can calculate how many calories you need in a day to lose weight or maintain weight.

Ideally you want your metabolic rate to be on the high side so you can burn more calories than you take in, leading to weight loss. Maintaining your weight means you take in the same amount of calories that you burn.

There are many ways to calculate your total energy expenditure (BMR plus physical activity) and numbers can vary greatly. There are also many good online software programs that will do that for you, where all you need to do is plug in your height, weight, and activity level. Some of these simply calculate calories, such as webmd.com or mayoclinic.com, others calculate BMI and calorie counts based on weight loss (if you want to lose 1 or 2 pounds a week) such as mynetdiary.com or caloriescount.com. I recommend checking out some of these sites—most are free but do require membership, and others charge a small fee and include other perks like food logs, reports, community, articles, and advice/tips from dietitians. See Appendix B for a fuller list of specific sites to check out. If you want a general ballpark figure use the following formula:

1. Divide your weight by 2.2 to get weight in kilograms.

2. Multiply this number (weight in kg) by 23 for women and 24 for men.

3. Add in a percent for physical activity, which usually runs:

   20 percent for sedentary adults (little or no exercise)

   30 percent for lightly active (exercise 1 to 3 times per week)

   40 percent for moderately active (3 to 5 times per week)

   If you are training for a marathon or sporting event or athlete, increase this percentage number even higher.

4. To lose weight, decrease your total caloric intake by 500 calories per day. Because there are 3,500 calories in one pound of fat, dropping your calorie intake 500 calories, while increasing exercise (increasing energy output), would yield a 1- to 2-pound weight loss per week. Although results may vary depending on how much you weigh from the start and activity level, this is about the level you want to be at. If you are a small person and have a low calorie level try not to drop below 1200 calories, in this case rather than decrease calories concentrate on increasing physical activity instead.

For example: if a woman weighed 150 pounds, divide 150 by 2.2 to get her kilogram weight: 68.

Next, take this number and multiply it by 23:

$68 \times 23 = 1,564$ (This is base caloric needs)

For a lightly active person, add 469 calories (30 percent of 1,564) to the base calorie number, giving her about 2,038 calories per day.

For a weight loss of 1 pound per week to occur she must decrease her caloric intake by 500 calories. Therefore, her calorie intake goal to lose weight would be:

$2,038 - 500 = 1,538$ calories per day

To speed weight loss to 2 pounds per week she would need to bump up physical activity rather than decrease any more calories. That's because cutting calories too low, below your BMR, shifts your body into starvation mode and lowers your metabolic rate. This also means you switch from a fat burner to a fat storer, as your body tries to conserve energy, making it really hard to lose weight. This is one reason why starvation diets don't work. You also run the risk of coming up short in essential vitamins and minerals.

Rather you want to eat well, eat frequently, and eat when you're hungry to avoid dropping your calories too low. At the same time you want to boost your metabolism to burn as many calories as you can at rest. What's the best way to do this? Exercise of course, but diet can enhance this effect.

> **GOOD MOVE**
>
> Although the best way to boost metabolism is to eat less and move more, there are some foods that burn more calories than others and should be included in your diet. These are caffeinated beverages (see Chapter 7); chili peppers; green tea; and lean, high-protein foods.

Breakfast Every Morning

When it comes to losing weight and burning fat there's one meal you don't want to miss and that's breakfast. Breakfast eaters are more likely to weigh less, have smaller middles, and consume fewer total daily calories than breakfast skippers. Furthermore, for "successful losers" (people who have lost weight and kept it off for more than a year), breakfast eating is a common characteristic and more often than not a regular daily ritual. So why is breakfast so important?

Big Returns at No Cost

After a good night's sleep and several hours of fasting, your body needs fuel to kick-start your metabolism and get you moving again. Your morning meal provides you with this much-needed energy, preventing you from going into famine mode and reducing cortisol levels, which gradually climbed during the night. It also ramps up your metabolism, switching you from fat storing to fat burning mode, and may give you a variety of healthy vitamins, minerals, and nutrients such as calcium, fiber, vitamins A and C, zinc, and iron—if you make a healthy breakfast choice.

Whether exercising, running off to work, or taking care of the kids, a good balance of protein, carbs, and good fats gives you the strength and endurance to make it through to lunch. But, eating first thing in the morning does more than just feed your body, it feeds your mind, too.

The brain uses more energy than any other organ in the body. Even though it makes up only 2 percent of our body weight, it uses about 20 percent of our total daily calories, primarily in the form of glucose. Eating breakfast gives you the calories you need to stay sharp, focused, and alert, improving concentration and performance. Children who eat breakfast behave better in school and have better cognitive function, attention spans, and memory skills than children who don't eat breakfast. And, these cognitive improvements are seen in adults as well.

RED FLAG

Don't wait more than a few hours from the time you get up to the time you put something in your stomach. If you do, rising cortisol levels will push you into famine mode, your metabolism will drop, and your body will begin conserving energy and fat. The best way to avoid this is to plan your breakfast ahead of time.

So what if you opt to skip this morning meal like nearly 40 percent of all adult Americans and even more (as much as 60 percent) of children and teens? Missing breakfast even once will yield these immediate results—your energy will fade quickly and you'll feel tired, weak, and lethargic; mentally you'll be out-of-sorts, foggy headed, lightheaded, and headachy. You'll also find it hard to concentrate and may become irritable and quick-tempered.

What's worse is how these effects cascade into a series of events that lead to poor eating habits throughout the day. Forced into starvation mode, your body will crave high-calorie, concentrated sweets and fats. Because you're hungry, you're more likely to give in to those cravings, grabbing a donut, pastry, or croissant, and because you haven't eaten since the night before you're also more likely to over indulge. Consequently, people who regularly skip breakfast actually tend to eat more during the day than people who eat breakfast. They also make poorer food choices. Long-term the stakes are high. People who forgo their morning meal …

- Are more likely to be overweight or obese (particularly around the middle).

- Are less likely to exercise regularly.

- Have higher rates of heart disease.

- Have higher rates of Type 2 diabetes.

- Are more likely to die of heart failure.

Zero In on Protein

So what should you eat for breakfast? While having a mocha grande coffee or grabbing a mega muffin is better than no breakfast at all and will stop you from going into starvation mode and lowering your metabolism, you should still think twice about what you eat since calories can add up quickly, resulting in you taking in 2 or even 3 times more calories than necessary. Poor breakfast choices like the one I mentioned will also set you up to crash and burn later on, as glucose levels spike and then quickly drop. The result is that you feel hungrier quicker. A bagel with cream cheese or butter is no better and may even be worse because it can be even higher in calories and sodium than sugary pastries, is highly refined, and contains few nutrients. Furthermore, it still won't satisfy you, leading to feelings of hunger not long after.

What's your best bet?

- **High-protein foods.** Make high-protein foods like eggs, greek yogurt, lean meats, fish, reduced-fat cheese, low-fat milk, and beans a priority during breakfast. Not only is protein good for your brain, your muscles, and your body (protein foods help lower insulin response and maintain blood sugar levels), they can also help you lose weight. A high-protein breakfast makes you feel full and satisfied hours after you've eaten, making it easier to stick to a weight-loss plan. Aim for 15 to 20 grams of protein for breakfast.

> **GOOD MOVE**
>
> Eat some eggs for breakfast. Eggs are considered the ideal protein food. One egg provides 6 grams of protein and 70–80 calories (one ounce of meat or poultry contains 7 grams of protein). It is low in saturated fat and is a good source of riboflavin, vitamin B_{12}, phosphorous, and selenium. Although most of the protein is found in the white part of the egg, don't throw out the yolk. It contains valuable nutrients that together (white and yolk) provide the "perfect protein."

- **Whole grains.** Whole grains provide the complex carbohydrates your body needs along with the fiber. High-fiber foods fill you up and contain plenty of B vitamins and minerals. Most of our whole grains are in the form of cereal, but beware of highly processed products loaded with sugar and artificial ingredients. Instead choose more natural cereals like oatmeal and whole-grain flakes. Also, cereal alone (even with milk) won't give you enough protein to keep you satisfied until lunch, so plan on filling in the holes by adding a high-protein food, such as a hard-cooked egg, to your meal.

- **Good fats.** One of these good fats—nuts, seeds, olives, and avocados—should be included in every meal. They're great for adding color, crunch, and taste. Although considered "good," beware of overdoing it—watch portion size, as you want to eat only small amounts. This is one case where you can easily get too much of a good thing, leading to weight gain.

- **Fruits and vegetables.** Fruits and/or vegetables are pretty much standard fare at breakfast and easy to add to many dishes like omelettes, cereals, and sandwiches. Choose whole fruits over juice.

WHAT'S NEW

Dieters who drink skim milk during breakfast experienced greater satiety and eat 200 calories less for lunch than dieters who drink a fruit drink for breakfast. This is likely due to the protein and the calcium in the milk.

Many people get stuck eating the same thing for breakfast every morning. They also have a traditional "breakfast food" mentality—meaning only certain foods should be eaten for breakfast. That's absolutely not true. Your morning meal can be anything you want it to be—from last nights' dinner to a fruit smoothie to a veggie-filled sandwich. When it comes to breakfast think outside the box and choose what you like. The best way to ensure you eat a good breakfast is to make it the night before. Here are a few morning meal ideas to get you started:

- Vegetable omelette wrapped in a whole-wheat tortilla with a glass of skim milk

- One cup of low-fat plain yogurt with fruit, nuts, and low-fat/low-sugar granola or dry cereal

- Peanut butter and jelly or tuna sandwich on whole-wheat bread with a pear

- One cup cooked oatmeal mixed with 1 tablespoon almond butter, 1 tablespoon yogurt, and any fresh or dried fruit

- One cup cooked red beans, salsa, one scrambled egg, and two slices avocado

- Yogurt and cottage cheese fruit smoothie mixed with 1 tablespoon flaxseed

Eat Every Three Hours

Now that you've taken care of breakfast it should be easy to spread out your calories throughout the day. Your total intake should consist of three main meals, 300 to 500 calories each, plus two substantial snacks, which should include some type of protein, fat, and carbohydrate. Think 1 tablespoon of peanut butter on 2 or 3 whole-grain crackers with an apple or low-fat string cheese, a small handful of almonds, or an orange.

So you don't go over your calorie quota, divide the number of calories you want to eat by 4. Then divide one of those numbers in half. This gives you three meals and two snacks (the smaller half numbers). So if you're on a 1,500-calorie diet, that would mean four eating occasions at 375 calories each. If you divide one of those in half that gives you two snacks, at 190 calories each plus breakfast, lunch, and dinner at 375 calories each.

Eating this way means you'll be eating every three hours with no longer than five hours between some type of meal or snack. Why? Regularly supplying your body with calories prevents sugar levels from dipping too low, resulting in fatigue and tiredness. It also prevents you from getting so hungry you overeat.

Re-Instituting the Family Dinner at Home

It's really worth it to try to eat dinner as a family at least five times a week. It's good for your belly fat loss because you're in control of the ingredients in your meal, and you create good examples for social interaction and support to manage stress. There are lots of other benefits of making family dinner a habit as well:

- Kids who eat dinner at home tend to eat more fruits and vegetables and less soda and fried foods.

- People who eat at home get more calcium, fiber, and iron in their diets.

- Teenagers who eat fewer than three dinners at home with family are two to three times more likely to have used marijuana, alcohol, and cigarettes than those who eat dinner together.

Unfortunately, many people don't put a priority on eating at home together. Only about 39 percent of non-Hispanic white adolescents eat dinner with their families at home, along with 40 percent of black and 54 percent of Hispanic adolescents.

And, this is even more prevalent in affluent urban areas where in many cases both parents work. Case in point, when my son was in sixth grade the teacher asked the children how many people eat dinner with their family at least five times a week. In a class of 24 children only my son raised his hand, and he was embarrassed! Although this may be an extreme example it brings home the point that as we get busier and busier, fewer families make time for eating together. If you want to improve your and your family's eating habits, you must be committed to eating nutritious food together, at least a few times a week.

WHAT'S NEW

Research shows kids who eat dinner with their families at home at least five nights per week are about 25 percent less likely to be overweight than kids who eat out more often. Seems like common sense, but it's important to take a look at how your family eats.

A Light but Satisfying Meal

Dinner is often a social meal, and this can make it too big. But it's also a great time to model making healthful, nutritious choices. Even if your family doesn't like vegetables, include a colorful array of them on the table and be sure and take a healthy portion of them—remember vegetables make great leftovers and can easily be added to omelettes, pastas, stir-fries, and whole-grain dishes. Rather than covering them up with butter and cheese (in the hopes of getting someone to try it), prepare these foods as you would like them and as recommended in some of the recipes included in this book. Use fresh herbs and interesting spices. This also allows you more versatility in using these vegetables in other recipes later on in the week.

Here are some other healthy dinner behaviors to keep you on track and feeling good about yourself and your family:

- **Get everyone involved.** Getting everyone involved in making dinner does two things: it improves the chances that the family will eat the meal—when you prepare something yourself you're more likely to eat it—and it takes quite a bit of workload off of you. If you want to add one more benefit, you can be content to know you're teaching your kids how to prepare a healthy meal.

- **Portion out plates and don't go back for seconds.** If losing weight is your goal, the best way to control portions and not overeat is to keep the serving platters off the table. Plate up portions for you and your family at the stove or on a separate counter. If someone wants seconds they have to physically get up to get it, a deterrent for overeating. This also gives you time to be more mindful of when you're full.

- **Try new things.** Broaden your and your family's culinary horizons by trying something new. This could be introducing your family to a new food, new cooking technique, or new ethnic cuisine. Keep things simple, don't try too many new things at once, and don't be discouraged if it doesn't turn out as you expected. Consider it an adventure in cooking. If you and your family like it you can incorporate it into your regular menu.

- **Make it fun.** Eating dinner together should be fun and enjoyable—a time to reconnect with loved ones and talk about your day. Don't get uptight if your family doesn't like your food or your meal doesn't go as planned. Everyone is not going to love every meal and every meal is not going to be a spectacular culinary achievement. Sometimes dinner ends up being fruit, cheese, and granola or crackers and that's okay—just smile, knowing cleanup will be a breeze.

What About After-Dinner Snacks?

Although there isn't a lot of evidence that eating a low-calorie dinner is a big boon to weight loss, there are many reasons to avoid eating *anything* after dinner. Nighttime snacking usually involves high-calorie foods with lots of fat. In one study, people who went to bed late ate twice as much fast food and half as many fruits and vegetables as those with earlier bedtimes. They also were more likely to drink full-calorie sodas and eat more total calories in a day. Consequently people who go to bed late and eat late at night have higher BMIs than those who go to bed earlier.

Poor food choices and eating more calories, however, isn't the only reason people who eat late at night tend to put on the pounds. Animal studies that fed mice identical diets but that ate at different times of day (daytime versus nighttime) found those who ate at night gained significantly more weight than the daytime eaters. While human studies are yet to be done, this does make sense. For thousands of years humans ate between sunrise to sunset. After sunset there was just no food around.

Taking a break from eating does something else, too. It allows your insulin and stress hormone levels to fall to their natural low points as you approach bedtime. Going to bed with cortisol and insulin activated by a round of nighttime eating is a surefire way to hold on to belly fat.

GOOD MOVE

You'll avoid a lot of extra calories, fat, and sweeteners if you simply make it a rule to stop eating after dinner. You'll also have a better appetite for breakfast!

The best way to avoid this problem is to simply make a rule: no eating after dinner or no eating after 7 P.M. Because people often consume food mindlessly, those who snack after dinner consume a lot more calories per day than people who call it quits when the dinner dishes are done. Here are some tips for making dinner lean and satisfying:

- Eat plenty of fiber with dinner. Fiber bulks up and helps you avoid feeling hungry.

- Get a good serving of protein at dinner time—protein is the most satiating macronutrient you can eat.

- Start a nighttime tea ritual. Find some nice herbal, caffeine-free teas and treat yourself to a nice cup before bed. Chamomile and other relaxing herb teas can be a great idea. Tea can also substitute as a satisfying "dessert."

- If you've shorted yourself on water during the day, you can remedy that situation by sipping on a water bottle during the evening. It's best to stop drinking about an hour before bedtime, though, to avoid having to get up to urinate when you're sleeping.

On this program, you'll be eating no more than a third of each day's calories for dinner (less if you plan on some substantial snacks). Eating this way will also give you more energy for your after-dinner movement—which helps with digestion. You'll also be less likely to have heartburn and reflux symptoms.

If you must nibble on something later in the evening, be sure it is a healthy snack which includes protein, carbohydrate, and fat and is no more than 200 calories, and *be sure and stop eating at least two hours before you go to bed.*

Don't Go to Bed Hungry or Full

Going to bed too full can end up in a restless sleep, feeling bloated and heavy, but going to bed hungry can be a problem, too. This can also disrupt your sleep and lead to a grumpy, stressful morning. You should feel pretty neutral about food when you go to bed, and ready to eat a good meal when you wake up.

While some people are forced to eat late at night because of work schedules, others may suffer from a specific condition called *nighttime-eating syndrome*. This syndrome is proving to be an important risk factor for being overweight. Nighttime eaters are more likely to be obese than people who don't eat after dinner. This kind of eating is also associated with a lower likelihood of being an exerciser, a higher likelihood of being depressed, and being more stressed than people who don't tend to eat at night.

DEFINITION

Nighttime-eating syndrome is recognized as a type of unhealthy eating that's characterized by eating more than 25 percent of your calories after a normal dinner time and/or getting out of bed to eat during the night at least three times per week.

Nighttime eating is usually a form of emotional eating. Most people who eat a lot at night report that they often feel stressed out, upset, or anxious. The foods that most night eaters consume are usually high in fat and carbohydrates—read, comfort foods. Other evidence that night eating is stress-related comes from studies that found women who tend to eat at night have measurably higher levels of stress hormones.

Get Enough Sleep

Going to bed late and waking up late is one thing, but being chronically sleep-deprived, meaning not getting enough sleep, is another. People who are sleep-deprived are at a higher risk of putting on the pounds.

Like late-night eaters, sleepiness can cause you to make poor food choices, grabbing a sugary food or caffeinated beverage to give yourself a jolt awake, and skip exercising, making it harder for you to lose weight. Shortchanging yourself on sleep upsets the natural balance of hormones responsible for telling us when to stop and start eating (the hormone that tells us to start eating increases while the one that tells us to stop decreases). At the same time our metabolism slows down. These are two key factors that lead to weight gain.

How much sleep is enough? On average we need about 7.5 to 8 hours of sleep a night. Sleep-deprivation usually falls into the range of 5 hours or less, but much of this depends on the individual.

WHAT'S NEW

Kids who get at least 10 hours of sleep per night and watch less than 2 hours of TV per day are about 40 percent less likely to be overweight than kids who don't share this lifestyle.

The Least You Need to Know

- Eat a high-protein breakfast packed with whole grains, fiber, good fats, and whole fruits and vegetables every day.
- To keep your metabolism high and prevent you from overeating you should eat three small meals a day with a mid-morning and mid-afternoon snack, or two mid-afternoon snacks if there is a big span between lunch and dinner.
- Making family dinners together not only provides a healthy meal for your loved ones but also fosters social interaction and family bonding.
- Make it a rule: don't eat after dinner.
- If you want to lose belly fat make sure you get eight hours of sleep a night.

On the Move

Exercise is essential for getting rid of any fat, but particularly stubborn belly fat. But, it's not about spot training or doing 100 sit-ups. Physical activity and exercise decrease stress, improve health, and help your mind as well as your body—all important for toning your tummy. To get rid of belly fat you need a combination of cardiovascular work and strength training to build muscle. The more muscle you have the faster your metabolism and the less likely you are to put on weight (and the more likely you are to lose weight).

If you don't know where to start, or even if you do, this part will tell you exactly what you need to do to slim down your stomach. This includes working out at the gym, playing sports, or simply doing a few exercises at home.

Move That Body to Lose That Belly

In This Chapter

- Exercise is great, but being physically active is essential
- The problem with sitting
- Being sedentary isn't just lack of exercise
- Physical activity busts stress

In this chapter, we're going to show you a bunch of ways to get your body moving. In Chapters 13 and 14, you'll find a variety of workouts that will get your metabolism revved up and help you burn off your belly faster. Exercise is important, but it should be part of a generally active lifestyle—one that maximizes walking, climbing stairs, and even standing, while minimizing sitting. Sedentary living is one of the biggest causes of belly fat, and the information in this chapter is going to help you move your body as much as you can.

What It Means to be Sedentary

Large survey research has shown that about 55 percent of adults don't get any physical activity beyond basic activities of daily living, and about 33 percent get none at all. That leaves only about 12 percent of American adults engaging in at least a moderate level of leisure time activity, so it's no wonder that we have such a staggeringly high prevalence of chronic diseases associated with too much fat, especially belly fat, in our country.

Our lack of exercise and physical activity isn't taxing only our bodies, however. Many studies have documented exercise's effectiveness as a treatment for mild to moderate depression—in fact, exercise has been shown to be as effective as antidepressant medication in some people. In addition, regular physical activity works to improve the bad moods that come with everyday stress. People who exercise regularly have lower rates of insomnia and anxiety, and they've also been shown to have higher levels of confidence and self-esteem. So exercise and activity are good for body, mind, and spirit!

Physical Activity and Exercise: What's the Difference?

The Centers for Disease Control and the American College of Sports Medicine recommend 30 minutes or more of moderate intensity physical activity every day. Examples of moderate intensity physical activity include walking briskly at about 3 to 4 miles an hour; general calisthenics such as push-ups, chin-ups, and sit-ups; and working around the house or garden. So what's the difference between *physical activity*, the hot new topic in the world of obesity prevention, and *exercise?*

WHAT'S NEW

Hunger and appetite are regulated by a large number of hormones, all but one of which work to suppress appetite. Ghrelin, secreted by the stomach when it's empty, is one of the few that actually increases appetite. Moderate physical exercise leads to reductions in the secretion of ghrelin.

Physical activity is the activity that's part of a person's daily life. Household, workplace, and lifestyle physical activity are three of the most common types. Physical activity basically includes any body movements produced by skeletal muscles that results in energy expenditure. Exercise, on the other hand, is defined as a form of physical activity that's planned, structured, repetitive, and done to improve at least one aspect of physical fitness such as strength, flexibility, or aerobic endurance.

To put it more simply, exercise is something a person does for 30 to 60 minutes at a time—and this is great, but it's not enough to keep belly fat at bay. Being physically active entails keeping your body moving consistently, as much as possible, all day long by walking, lifting, carrying, and standing. By keeping yourself moving, you keep your muscles switched on and burning calories.

The Health Hazards of Sitting

The latest research into the scourge of physical inactivity in Americans has focused on the dangers of too much sitting. Stop for a moment and ask yourself, "how many hours a day do I spend sitting down?" Don't forget to include time spent driving in your car, sitting at your desk, watching TV, and working at your computer. If the total amounts to six hours or more per day, you may be putting your health and your belly at great risk—simply because you don't spend enough time up on your feet.

"Sedentary behavior" is not a synonym for "not exercising," but is rather a lifestyle pattern marked by prolonged hours of physical inactivity such as sitting. Recently, a new field of human health studies has emerged, called *inactivity physiology*. Scientists in this field have found that sitting down is a somewhat unnatural human behavior that causes dramatic shifts in your physiology. These shifts include significant increases in blood glucose levels. As we've seen, chronically elevated blood sugar leads to elevated insulin, which in turn promotes the collection of belly fat. People who sit a lot are more likely to lose bone density and muscle tissue as they age. As you lose muscle tissue, you lose the ability to burn energy efficiently and you're more likely to build up fat, especially in your belly.

 DEFINITION

Inactivity physiology focuses on the health consequences of sedentary behavior as something distinct from the health consequences of not exercising.

Here are some astonishing facts from the research on sitting and health:

- People with sitting jobs have twice the rate of cardiovascular disease as people with standing or walking jobs.

- As soon as you sit down, calorie burning drops to about 1 calorie per minute.

- The enzymes in your skeletal muscles that help break down fat and keep low-density lipoprotein (LDL) levels low reduce their activity by as much as 90 percent as soon as you take a seat.

- After two hours of sitting, high-density lipoprotein (HDL) levels drop by around 20 percent and stay down until you get up and start moving around again. Remember that HDL is the healthy form of cholesterol, and the more you have, the better.

Although I would be the last person to discourage you from going to the gym for a good workout three or four times a week, I can't deny the convincing evidence that this simply isn't enough to avoid belly fat and the health consequences of physical inactivity. A person who goes out and gets that 30 to 45 minutes of physical activity a day is doing something good, that's true. However if this person then sits down to drive around, work at a computer or other desk type job all day, eat meals, and watch TV at the end of the day, he may actually spend up to 90 percent of his waking hours sitting down. Ironically, by most definitions, you could call this person "physically active," but you'd be overlooking the drastic and unfortunate negative effects of all that chair time.

What inactivity physiology is showing us is that sitting down too much is not the same as not getting enough exercise. For this reason, the latest recommendations, based on the most reliable and recent research, should be that every person should aim to spend fewer than six or seven hours in a chair every single day.

If you have a job that demands you sit at a desk all day, don't despair. Getting up and moving around, even for only a few minutes each hour, reactivates your leg muscles and keeps their metabolic fires burning. If you work at a computer, consider setting its clock to chime every hour, reminding you to get up and walk around or stretch for 3 to 5 minutes.

You can spend your breaks and lunchtime on your feet to avoid the sluggish effects of sitting too long. You don't need to work up a sweat, you just need to move. You can probably think of other ideas to get yourself moving, like going to speak to colleagues in person instead of sending an email or going to pick up your mail instead of waiting for it to be delivered.

Inactivity Physiology: The Nitty Gritty

After a few hours of sitting, the most important change in physiology is what happens in your skeletal muscles. Skeletal muscles contain an enzyme called lipoprotein lipase (LPL). This enzyme is responsible for pulling fat out of your blood and into muscles so they can use that fat as fuel. This enzyme particularly likes to take up LDL particles, and as we've seen, LDL is one of the most dangerous forms of cholesterol when it occurs in levels that are higher than normal.

After seven or so hours of sitting, the LPL in the skeletal muscles decreases its activity by 75 to 90 percent. Why does this happen? The answer is simple—if you're not using your muscles, they're not going to be burning energy, so they won't be taking net energy. If LPL is not sucking cholesterol out of your bloodstream so your muscles can use it, the cholesterol stays in the blood, and levels tend to rise. As we saw in Chapter 3, when LDL levels are too high for too long, they can begin to collect in the arteries that feed the heart and the brain and contribute to the formation of heart attack– and stroke-causing plaque.

And adults aren't the only ones who sit around too much. Children obsessed with video games, television, and texting also spend way too much time sitting. In children, prolonged sitting increases the odds of being overweight or obese and developing diabetes. In Canada, newly published guidelines for children's health say no more than 25 percent of a child's day should be spent sitting. Basically, that means that after a child is done with his or her school day, he or she needs to be physically active right up until bedtime.

RED FLAG

Sitting down for several hours a day isn't dangerous only for adults. Children in North America spend an average of 8.6 hours a day being sedentary.

The Benefits of Physical Activity

Consistent physical activity is great for fat loss, especially belly fat loss. It's also a highly effective way to manage stress. Basically, being stressed out repeatedly throughout the day keeps cortisol levels high, leading to the release of sugar and fat into your blood in order to support the activity of your skeletal muscles so you can deal with an imminent threat.

Physical activity stimulates your muscles to use that extra fat and sugar as fuel. It can also suppress stress's effects on your blood pressure, and have positive effects on your mood and your ability to think clearly.

WHAT'S NEW

Exercise physiologists are discovering the important role that skeletal muscle plays in managing blood sugar and insulin levels. Muscles that get a lot of activity all day will stay hungry for sugar to replenish their glycogen stores. Muscles that don't work have no need to take up glucose for rebuilding glycogen, so they will shut down their insulin receptors to keep glucose out. This can eventually develop into insulin resistance, a precursor to Type 2 diabetes.

Physical Activity Leads to Stress Resilience

Studies of people who are physically active compared to those who are not has shown that the physically active have a less pronounced nervous system and endocrine response to acute psychological stressors; that is, they have less *cardiovascular reactivity*. This means simply that when a physically active person is presented with a challenge in his or her daily life, he or she won't have as much of a heart rate and blood pressure response as someone who is sedentary.

DEFINITION

Cardiovascular reactivity describes the elevations in heart rate and blood pressure that happen whenever you get stressed out.

High levels of cardiovascular reactivity are associated with an increased likelihood of dying of a heart attack or stroke. This is most likely due to mechanical damage done to your blood vessels when blood pressure gets too high and the repeated energy depletion of your heart muscle when such demands are placed on it, especially when you're out of shape.

It's also been found that stress has a smaller impact on immune function in people who are physically active than in people who are sedentary. In a way you can think of regular physical activity as a way to "train" for the stresses of everyday life. It seems that bodily movement, whether it's standing instead of sitting, walking instead of riding, or any other everyday physical activity you can think of is a fundamental way of staying resilient to stress.

Being Active Helps Your Mind

In general, people who are active reap many psychological and emotional benefits as a result of their physical exertions. Physically active people have been found to have less depression and bad moods than sedentary people. Being active has also been linked to better cognitive skills, creative thinking, social interactions, and stress management.

Being physically active helps keep your moods on the sunny side, apparently by helping keep your brain's production of serotonin at normal levels. Serotonin is known as your natural antidepressant, and levels are often low in people who are depressed. Regular physical activity and exercise seems to stimulate serotonin production, which probably explains why exercise has been shown to be as effective a treatment for mild to moderate depression as the drugs frequently prescribed for this condition.

GOOD MOVE

In addition to helping to elevate mood, serotonin also works to keep your appetite under control and suppress nonhunger-related eating. So next time you're in a bad mood and feel like grabbing a donut, try taking a walk or dancing around your living room for a few minutes. Chances are you'll feel better and forget all about that belly bloating "treat."

Getting Active, Starting Now

The beautiful part of our new understanding of the science of physical activity and sedentary physiology is that it's not as complicated as we once believed. What we are beginning to understand is that the key to staying lean and healthy is not to carve out an hour every day to go to the gym or an exercise class. Now before I continue, let me make myself clear: these are all good activities and definitely will help you be leaner and healthier. Regular exercise is going to be part of your belly fat program, and will hasten your fat loss. But it's only part of the story. The best bang for your belly fat loss buck is going to be finding as many ways as possible to be either standing or walking all day long.

I'm going to offer some ideas for getting more physical activity into your life, but I also leave it to you to find ways to fit this into your own unique lifestyle. If you work in an office at a desk all day, you'll need to find ways to get out of your chair on a regular basis. If you're a stay-at-home mom, this might be easier to do but may require some determination and thought. The bottom line is that whoever you are, you can almost certainly spend more time each day using your muscles and moving your body.

Stand Up to Be Lean

We've discussed the dangers of sitting. Even if you work at a desk all day, that doesn't mean you have to always be sitting. If you must sit in a chair, set an alarm on your watch or computer to remind you to get up at least once an hour and stand or walk for at least five minutes. This will instantly recharge the muscles of your legs and get them active again. Make it a rule to stand up to talk on the phone, or to open your mail. Keep looking for things you can do standing that you normally do sitting, and you'll be able to shave lots of sitting time out of your day.

Many experts in the health and wellness field, including myself, have done away with their desk chairs. All the recent evidence of the evils of sitting has motivated me and many others to use a standing desk. As an author, I spend hours a day at my computer, and that used to mean hours of sitting. No more! I'm on my feet all day, and I no longer get the stiff shoulders and stagnant feeling that my desk chair used to give me. A standing desk is easy to devise, and you can even buy a ready-made one at IKEA and other furniture stores.

GOOD MOVE

Buy or make a standing desk. A standing desk is one that's high enough that you can type or write at while standing up. It may feel strange at first, but most people who use standing desks say they feel more energetic and less stiff after a day's work.

If you want to watch television, stand up and fold laundry or do some other activity while you're watching if you've been sitting all day. It's easy to limit chair time if you start to look for opportunities throughout your day to choose to stand instead.

Take Steps to a Flat Belly

It can be pretty simple to get more steps into your day. Try to limit the use of your car if you live in an area where shops and other resources are nearby. If they're a little out of reach, consider taking public transportation instead of driving when you have time. Park your car far from the grocery store entrance and save the close parking spots for the elderly and infirm. You can also ditch your car altogether and use your bike to run errands whenever possible.

We've all heard the admonition to "take the stairs," and you'd do well to follow it. You can even challenge yourself to even greater heights. Make it a rule to always take the stairs if you're going two flights up or less. Then add one. Then another. I have a colleague who eschews the elevator and walks the stairs up to her eighth floor apartment after work each day. This is a great idea, because you can burn up to 300 calories in 30 minutes of walking up stairs. The research shows that all the physical activity you do in a day counts. So if you walk up a few stairs here and there, the energy burn can really add up.

If you want to see how many steps you really take in a day, invest in a pedometer. The generally agreed upon goal for optimal benefit from walking is to take 10,000 steps a day. A pedometer will tell you how much you're walking now, and how close you can get to the 10K ideal.

> **GOOD MOVE**
>
> A pedometer is a small device you strap to your waistband that counts the number of steps you take every day. Many studies have shown that wearing a pedometer increases exercise and walking activity, leading to significant weight loss even without making major changes to eating habits.

There are so many ways to get more walking into your daily life. Avoid drive-thrus whenever you can—and they're everywhere from the bank to the pharmacy. Promise yourself a couple of short strolls each day. In fact, a couple 10-minute walks per day will be part of your belly fat prescription. Ideally you'll gradually lengthen one of these walks to 20 or 30 minutes to get the maximum benefit. At the airport, use layovers to get extra steps in by avoiding the moving sidewalks. Bypass the fast-food restaurants and grab an apple and some nuts at one of the shops. Take a walk while you enjoy your snack, and be sure to drink some water to stay hydrated.

Hunter-gatherers didn't just walk, they also did plenty of lifting and carrying. You can imitate them by getting active around the house. Cleaning house, gardening, and home improvement projects all involve good whole-body muscular activity. Try to look at these things, as well as carrying groceries and other "chores," as opportunities to activate your muscles and fire up your metabolism.

The Least You Need to Know

- An important step toward losing belly fat is to minimize the amount of time you spend sitting.
- Increasing physical activity keeps stress at bay, normalizes blood chemistry, elevates mood, and accelerates belly fat loss.
- Increase metabolic activity in your skeletal muscles by standing and walking as much as possible throughout the day.

Workouts That Work

In This Chapter

- Exercise has physical and mental benefits
- Simple ways to make exercise part of your life
- While your belly shrinks, flatten it with core work
- Strong abs aren't just about looking good

By now it's common knowledge that exercise is a vital part of losing excess body fat and keeping it off. Study after study has demonstrated that without exercise, a weight-loss program may produce short-term results, but long-term maintenance is nearly impossible without incorporating regular exercise into your lifestyle.

More than just weight maintenance or weight loss, exercising regularly has many other benefits as well. It can stave off chronic disease, increase longevity, keep you mentally fit, reduce stress, and improve your quality of life. How? Read on and we'll explain each of these benefits in detail in this chapter. We'll also give you tips on how to get started leading a full, active life. Move your body on a regular basis and you'll quickly see results—changes in your mind, your body, and your belly.

Exercise Helps You Live Longer and Better

There are scads of studies out there showing that people who get regular exercise tend to have lower rates of cardiovascular disease and to live longer. Most of these studies focus on aerobic exercise like running, fitness walking, and biking.

Aerobic exercise is great for improving the health of your heart and lungs and keeping your energy levels high. It's also a great way to relieve the tension of a stressful day. There are two major ways that getting regular exercise can benefit you: physiological and psychological.

Physiological Benefits of Exercise

Let's take a look at the physiological benefits of exercise and activity. They include the following:

- Enhanced cardiorespiratory fitness

- Increased energy levels throughout the day

- More complete utilization of fat and sugars in the blood, keeping levels within normal limits

- Reduction in muscle tension, leading to less fatigue

- Reduction in immune system inflammation

- Less extreme insulin responses to eating a given amount of sugar and other simple carbohydrates

- Decreased risk of age-related cognitive losses such as dementia and memory loss

Inflammation is a very important risk factor for the development of cardiovascular disease. While losing weight is generally good for you in that it can reduce your inflammation levels, it's been found that whether or not you reap the full effects of this benefit depends on the method you use to lose the weight. In most research, people who use dieting alone tend to have an increase in their inflammatory markers as they lose weight. In contrast to this, people who use exercise and diet to lose weight tend to show marked reductions in overall inflammation. Even if you don't lose weight, regular physical activity and exercise helps cool the fires of inappropriate chronic inflammation.

WHAT'S NEW

An exciting new area of research has revealed yet another benefit of regular physical activity and exercise: staving off age-related dementia, brain shrinkage, and memory loss. We've long known that sedentary people experience more rapid losses of cognitive abilities as they age when compared to active people. It appears that being active maintains healthy levels of several compounds made by and for the brain, such as insulin-like growth factor (IGF-1) and brain-derived neurotropic factors (BDNF). Loss of brain power seems to parallel falling levels of these molecules, and being active appears to keep them relatively plentiful.

Psychological Benefits of Exercise

There are three basic theories about why exercise is good for stress. The first is the mastery hypothesis, which states that you feel good about yourself when you're active because you've taken a positive, active step toward better health and vitality. The second theory is the distraction hypothesis, which posits that exercise is a good way to get away from your troubles for a while. Finally, it's thought that exercise done in group settings like team sports and fitness classes serves our inherent need for social interaction and cooperation. Whatever the reason, there are many good reasons to keep your body moving and even push yourself a little harder than usual on a regular basis.

Exercise has other effects on brain chemistry, too. It's associated with release of dopamine during and between active periods. Dopamine is the neurotransmitter most commonly associated with great moods, pleasure, and happiness. In fact, many drugs of abuse have their effects by stimulating dopamine production in the brain, which is probably why they can be so addictive. You can get a milder, more natural "high" with exercise.

WHAT'S NEW

While it's true that almost any kind of exercise can help reduce stress, a recent study found that the types of exercise that do it best tend to have four specific characteristics: being aerobic, noncompetitive, predictable, and repetitive. Examples of this would include swimming, vigorous yoga, walking, and dancing.

Endorphins, your brain's natural opiates, are also released during exercise, especially if it's strenuous. This is thought to be the cause of the "runner's high" so many exercisers experience. Endorphins also block pain signals and cortisol release by the adrenals, making exercise less arduous and contributing to its stress-busting effects.

How to Become an Exerciser

Your flat belly program includes hiking up your daily dose of physical activity. As we saw in the previous section, the more routine physical activity you build into your schedule, the more quickly and efficiently you'll lose your belly fat. I also recommend that you layer an exercise routine on top of your new increased level of physical activity to speed up the rate at which you'll lose your belly fat.

The best way to do this is to add at least 30 to 40 minutes a day of moderate exercise to your schedule on 5 to 7 days every week. Brisk walking is a perfect way to get this exercise. It's free, you can do it anywhere at any time, it's low impact, and it helps keep your stress physiology under control. As I mentioned, if you're not already used to exercising you can start with two 10-minute strolls per day, and gradually work up to at least one brisk 30-minute walk a day.

In Chapter 11, we discussed the timing of eating and moving. With this information in mind, we recommend that you take your longer walk in the first 30 minutes after dinner. This will help you clear your bloodstream of sugar and insulin and get your muscles warm and tension free as you relax into your evening. If you're so inclined, you can add some more strenuous activities to your routine to really melt away your belly.

Jogging, Running, and Beyond

It's a common fallacy that running a mile burns the same number of calories as walking a mile. Conventional wisdom holds that running burns about 100 calories a mile, and because you do the same amount of work moving your body weight a mile when you walk, that should burn 100 calories, too. This isn't true, however. The best way to determine how many calories are burned in any given physical activity is to see how much oxygen is being consumed while you're doing it.

Recent research has shown that both men and women burn about 40 percent more calories running than walking the same distance. So you can see that running for a certain amount of time can burn a lot more calories than walking for that same period of time. First of all, you burn more calories per mile, and secondly, you can cover more ground when running for half an hour than walking. You can use the following table to calculate the number of calories burned in either running or walking, based on your body weight.

Activity	Net Calorie Burn/Mile
Running	0.63 × your weight in pounds
Walking at 3 to 4 mph	0.30 × your weight in pounds

Running isn't for everyone, however. If you're older than 50, you should have your cardiovascular fitness level tested by your doctor before you begin a running program. This is a good idea for you no matter what your age if you need to lose more than 20 pounds or have been sedentary for a long time. If you have problems with your joints, specifically your ankles, knees, hips, or lower back, it would be wise to consider a different activity that involves putting less strain on your joints. Two great alternatives to running are working out on an *elliptical trainer* and rebounding. Training on an elliptical machine can burn almost as many calories per hour as running does, with none of the risks of high-impact running.

DEFINITION

An **elliptical trainer** is a piece of exercise equipment found in most gyms and available for home use. It's a stationary machine that has two foot pads to stand on, and sometimes moving handles as well. The motion is similar to cross-country skiing, but also has elements of jogging and stair climbing.

Rebounding is jumping on a mini trampoline. This activity is fun and certainly gets your heart rate up. In addition there is evidence that rebounding helps stimulate your lymphatic circulation, which is great for clearing the toxins released during a fat-loss program. The typical mini trampoline used for rebounding is about 3 feet in diameter and 9 inches high. Using a rebounder, you can jump up and down to your heart's content without worrying about doing any damage to the joints of your lower body.

Jump on a Bike

Another great way to get strenuous exercise is riding a bike. Whether you choose to ride a stationary bike or get on one outside, you can derive great cardiovascular and fat-loss benefits. The quadriceps on the front of your thighs and the hamstrings on the back of your thighs are the largest muscles in your body. Working those muscles regularly by cycling is a great way to soak up any extra fat or sugar in your blood.

If you've never cycled for fitness, you'll find that it's not hard to get started. In the gym, you can choose between a standard bike or a recumbent bike. Both will give you a good workout. When deciding between them, consider your core. You'll work your back and abdominal muscles harder on the upright bike, hastening your way to a firmer torso. So unless you have a lot of lower back pain and strain, go for the upright every time. The newer bikes have all kinds of programs that vary the intensity of your workout.

Even more fun than cycling inside is taking a ride out in nature. Road bikes tend to have thin wheels and between three and more than a dozen gears. You can keep it very simple with an old-school, three-speed bike with regular pedals, or you can get a bike with toe clips and multiple gears. If you live in an area with a lot of hills, you'll probably prefer riding a bike that has a series of very low gears.

GOOD MOVE

A great way to add intensity and fun to your bike workout is to try a spin class at a gym. These classes are led by trained instructors and usually include music to keep you going. The bikes are designed to allow full control over the resistance and difficulty of your workout, so you can go at your own level. It's estimated that you can burn up to 500 calories in a one-hour class.

Mountain biking has grown in popularity in recent years. A good mountain bike will have shock absorbers under the seat and beneath the handlebars. Mountain bikes have fat knobby tires for good traction on all types of surfaces. I like mountain biking because out on the trails I don't have to worry about cars, and it's becoming ever easier to find fun, beautiful trails to ride on. If you haven't ridden a bike for a while, now might be a good time to rediscover the childlike joy of whizzing along on two wheels.

The Sporting Life

You don't have to be a super athlete to enjoy a sport. Anything to get you outside and moving around is going to help you lose belly fat and feel less stress. It's simple to add some kind of sport to your lifestyle. You can install a badminton net in your backyard, or invest in a croquet set. Even horseshoes can be a good form of exercise. The same caveats I mentioned with respect to running should be considered if you're thinking of taking up a more strenuous sport like soccer or basketball. Whatever you choose to do, pick a sport that's best suited to you physically and remember that it's all about having fun and enjoying the company of family and friends.

Visible Results: Core Work for a Flat Belly

Let's get one thing clear: doing core and abdominal exercises will not get rid of belly fat. The only reliable way to do that is the combination of eating style, physical activity, and stress management we explain in this book. That said, there's a strong case to be made for making some type of core workout a part of your weekly routine.

There are so many benefits to having strong abdominal and back muscles that we had to include a core workout in this program. If you're already groaning, expecting us to demand 100 sit-ups or crunches every day, cheer up! What we're suggesting is a series of concentrated, effective movements that, if practiced regularly, will enhance your belly fat loss program by making your abdomen firmer and flatter.

Strong Abs, Flatter Belly

One reason why most effective core workouts include a variety of exercises is that your belly has several different muscles. The one most people are aware of (and the foundation of "six pack abs") is the rectus abdominus, which runs vertically from the pubic bone to your sternum.

Many exercises, like standard sit-ups, tend to work only the rectus abdominus, neglecting the other muscle groups that are essential for good posture and a trimmer waist. The external and internal oblique muscles wrap around your sides, and help with twisting and sideways bending. They're important stabilizers for all types of physical activity.

GOOD MOVE

Unlike the muscles of your arms and legs, which need a day of rest between workouts to repair and build more fibers, your abdominal muscles can be worked every day with a moderate core program.

The deepest muscle layer in your abdominal wall is the transversus abdominus, which wraps horizontally around your belly, helping you breathe and stabilizing your spine. A strong transversus functions somewhat like a corset, keeping you in good alignment and more resilient to trips and stumbles.

Beyond Vanity: The Benefits of Strong Abs

For many of us, the prospect of a trim, firm tummy is plenty of motivation to do core exercises that work. But the benefits of having strong, flexible abdominal and back muscles go beyond the aesthetics of your form. Here are three documented benefits of getting your abs in shape:

1. **Better posture:** A sure sign of a weak torso is slouchy posture, which limits the volume of your breathing and contributes to low back pain. Strong ab and back muscles will hold you up straight naturally—which will make you look thinner!

2. **Fewer injuries:** A strong core is associated with better balance and fewer falls, because these muscles help you maintain stability in your hips and pelvis, and keep you steady if you start to stumble.

3. **Relief from and prevention of back pain:** Contrary to popular belief, the best treatment for low back pain isn't bed rest, but mild to moderate exercise that includes stretching and strengthening back and abdominal muscles.

A Basic Daily Core Routine

Here is a series of five core-strengthening *Pilates* exercises that you can do in about ten minutes. We recommend that you try these exercises and aim to do a few of them every day. As you lose the fat from inside and out of your belly, your results will be visible more quickly if you're also tightening your waist.

DEFINITION

Pilates is a system of exercises developed by Joseph Pilates, originally to help children with asthma breathe more easily by strengthening back and stomach muscles. Over time, his system of core work became popular among professional dancers and athletes. Today, there are about 14,000 Pilates instructors in the United States, who offer training in one-on-one and group formats.

If you haven't done much abdominal work or other exercise for a while, start slowly. Try one rep of each exercise, and work up to 8 to 10 reps each time you do your core work. If you ever feel pain or strain in your lower back while doing these movements, simply relax out of it and breathe deeply.

Don't be discouraged if you find these movements hard to do at first—that just means you have so much more to gain! The abdominal muscles tend to strengthen quickly, so you'll probably be surprised by how many reps you can do after a couple weeks of practice.

Here is your basic core workout:

1. Breathing

Seated in a comfortable position on your yoga mat or in a chair, sit up tall. From here, gently place both hands on your belly and close your eyes. Shift your attention to your breath. As you inhale through your nose, allow your belly to soften, as your ribcage, chest, and belly expand. Draw your breath into your hands on your belly. As you exhale through your mouth, engage your core by pulling your belly button back toward your spine.

Count to 5 slowly as you inhale, softening your belly and expanding your torso. Count to 5 slowly as you exhale, pulling your belly button in and engaging your core. Repeat this intentional slow and steady breath 12 times.

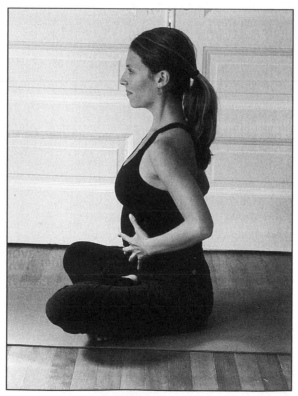

Make sure you fully relax your belly muscles to allow for a full breath.

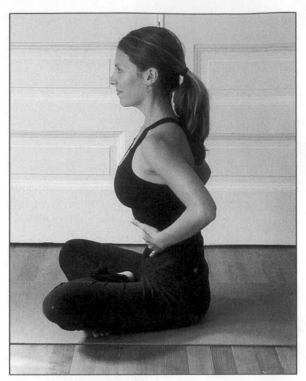

Use your abdominal muscles to gently push all the air out.

2. Boat Pose

Seated in the middle of your yoga mat with your legs bent and feet planted slightly wider than your hips on the mat, bring your hands underneath your knees. Shift your weight back so that you are balancing on your tailbone. From here, lift your legs up off the floor until they are parallel with the floor. Your knees are bent. Lengthen your spine and lift your chest up toward the ceiling.

Pull your lower belly in. When you are balanced, release your hold of the knees and keep the legs in the same position, suspended in the air parallel to your yoga mat. Hold here and breathe. Hold for 5 to 10 breaths. To release out, simply place your feet back down on the yoga mat.

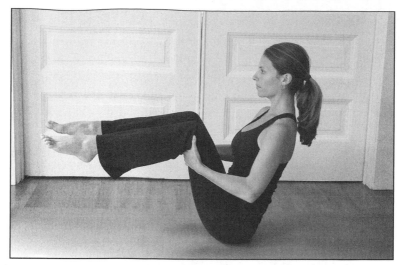

Use a good grip on your legs to support your back in this pose until your abs are strong enough to do most of the work.

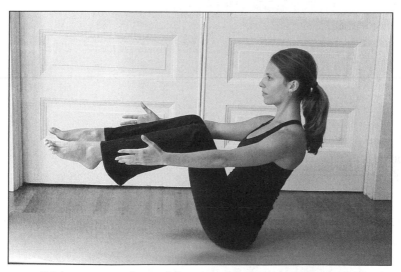

Make sure your abs are fully engaged to protect your lower back.

3. Roll Down and Crunches

Step 1: Begin by sitting on your yoga mat with your knees bent in front of you, and your feet placed in front of you on the yoga mat hip-width distance apart (knees are pointing up toward the ceiling). Extend your arms forward as if you were reaching for something in front of you. From here keep reaching forward as you slowly roll down onto your back. Roll down until your lower back is flat on the floor but your upper back and shoulders are still lifted; you are still reaching forward.

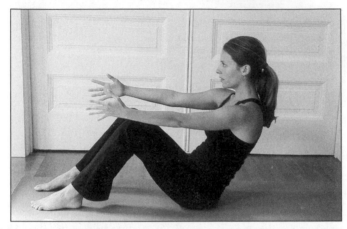

Roll down as slowly and deliberately as you can, and stop if you feel any discomfort in your lower back.

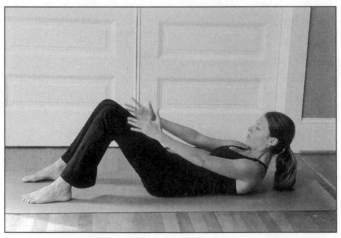

Support your neck by interlocking your fingers behind it if you feel fatigued.

Step 2: Stay here (shoulders still lifted), and as you inhale for a count of four, pick up your right leg, set it down on the mat as you exhale, again for a count of four. Inhale for four counts, picking up your left leg, and exhale for four counts, as you set it down. Then pick up both legs as you inhale for four. Exhale for four and set your feet down. Inhale and straighten your legs up to the ceiling. Stay here for a couple breaths and reach forward toward the front of your mat, shoulders lifted.

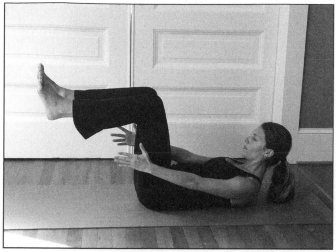

Use your whole core to support this pose—back, side, and upper and lower abs.

Step 3: Keep the legs extended up to the ceiling. (You can bend the knees if it is too intense of a stretch for your hamstrings.) Bring your hands behind your head, elbows wide so you cannot see them. Inhale and slowly release your head to the floor; as you exhale lift up slowly, engaging the core by pressing the lower back into the floor and lifting the shoulders up. Continue for 15 repetitions.

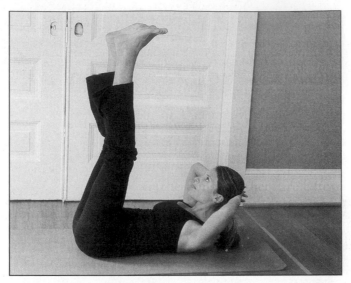

Be sure not to crunch your neck by focusing on keeping your head looking straight up at the ceiling.

4. Forearm Plank

Start in table top position on the hands and knees. From here, bring your forearms down to the yoga mat and extend the hands forward with your arms parallel to each other (your arms should look like a number 11 pointing to the front of your yoga mat). Elbows should be shoulder distance apart. Spread your fingers wide. When the arms are set up, extend your legs back, tuck your toes underneath, and press back into your heels coming into a forearm plank position. Make sure that your hips are low. Shoulders need to remain stacked directly over your elbows the entire time to ensure proper strengthening in the joints. (If you have lower back problems, you can slightly lift the hips in the air to release strain in the lower back.)

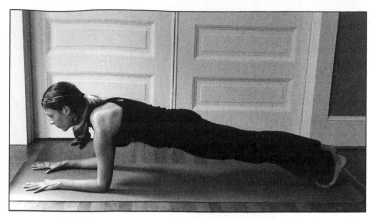

This is a great move that engages your entire core.

As you hold here, breathe, using the same breath that we used in Step 1 of these exercises. As you inhale let the belly soften. As you exhale engage the core and pull the belly button in toward the spine. Here in forearm plank feel everything draw in toward the center of your belly. Hold here for 10 slow and steady breaths. If this is too much, start by holding the plank for only one breath and build up.

5. Forearm Plank with Leg Lift

If you would like to add on to your forearm plank, you can practice lifting one leg at a time while still keeping the body in plank. As you inhale, lift the right leg 4 inches straight up off the floor; keep the foot flexed as you continue to press back into the heel of the lifted leg. Hold for a count of five. Exhale as you set the foot down. Repeat on the other side. Repeat as many times as you can, shifting from one leg to the other. Make sure that you are moving slowly and with control. Remember, as you inhale, lift the leg, and as you exhale, set the foot down. Repeat three times on each side, six times total, adding more repetitions as you get stronger.

At the beginning, it may be difficult to lift your leg while in plank. If this is true for you, substitute lifting your leg with simply bending it to 90 degrees, then straightening it, alternating as above. When you can do six reps on each side, advance to lifting your leg instead.

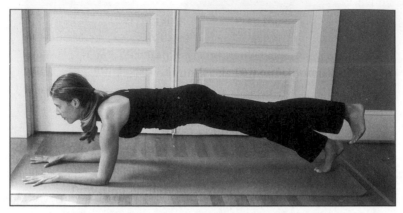

This is a fantastic way to tone your butt and lower back.

6. Forearm Plank with Knee to Elbow

If the leg lifts were no problem continue to add on in your forearm plank by first lifting the right leg and then as you exhale, bend the knee, pulling the knee toward the right elbow. Remember to keep your hips low, even as they want to lift. Imagine if you were crawling under a fence and you had to stay low. After you bring the knee to the elbow, inhale and then extend the leg back and exhale as you set the foot down. Switch to the other side. Repeat three times on each side, six times total, adding more repetitions as you get stronger.

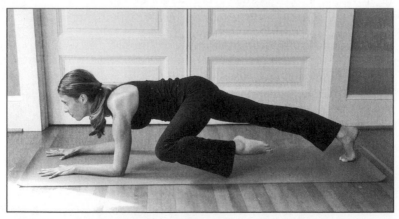

This is a very advanced move that provides an excellent workout for your oblique muscles.

Remember it is not specifically what you do but rather how you do it. In all of the listed exercises, make sure that your core is doing the work. Keep your jaw relaxed and neck long and straight. Lengthen your spine and pull your abdomen in tight. Move with control and use your breath (breathing in through your nose and out through your mouth) to deepen the pose.

These moves are very similar to the ones you can learn in a Pilates-based class, so if they're unfamiliar to you, try picking up a Pilates-based abdominal workout DVD. Better yet, try a class!

The Least You Need to Know

- Exercise for at least 30 minutes a day, at least 5 days a week, to lose that belly fat and keep it off.
- Keep your motivation up by incorporating things you enjoy into your workouts.
- Work your abdominal muscles every day to flatten your belly.

Build Muscle to Shrink Your Waist

In This Chapter

- Maintaining your muscles helps you burn fat
- Weight training builds muscles
- Strength training without weights
- Doing a simple weight routine at home or the gym

So far, we've talked about the fat-burning power of aerobic exercise and encouraged you to get your heart pumping with a brisk walk, jog, or bike ride on most, if not all, days a week. Now, we're going to explain why adding any type of muscle or strength training to your weekly schedule will get you closer to your goal of a trim, flat belly much faster than doing cardio alone.

Although it's true that doing aerobic exercise is great for heart health and is an important tool in fat loss, it generally only increases your metabolic rate while you're doing it, and for a little while afterward. On the other hand, adding muscle to your frame through strength training pays off twice—you burn calories while you're doing it, and the added muscle tissue on your body burns more calories per minute (all the time) than fat.

Skeletal Muscle and Belly Fat

Every time you eat, you're taking in energy in the form of fat and carbohydrates. These components of food are broken down into molecules like fatty acids and glucose that your cells can use for fuel. If your body is active, you'll tend to burn most of the fuel you take in. If you're sedentary or tend to overeat, there will most likely be excess fuel on board that gets stored as fat.

The average American adult loses about a quarter pound of muscle each year after the age of 40 unless he does regular strength training. As you lose muscle tissue, you lose your most voracious consumer of calories, leading to a drop in your basal metabolic rate. This is why so many people tend to gain weight as they age.

More Muscle, Faster Metabolism

About 80 percent of the energy in food is used by your body to maintain the function of your cells and organs. About 20 percent of the energy your body needs is consumed by your skeletal muscles. Unlike other tissues in your body, skeletal muscle is a very inefficient energy consumer, meaning that it takes more calories per hour to power active muscles than to maintain fat and other tissues.

WHAT'S NEW

Weight loss through caloric restriction alone has been shown to cause loss of muscle as well as fat. Studies have shown that weight training while losing weight prevents loss of muscle.

What this means to you is that if you keep your food intake constant but gradually add more muscle to your body, you'll burn up more energy every day, leaving little or no energy left over to store as fat.

Building Muscle to Age Well

Muscle building doesn't just keep you thin. It also helps stave off many of the common complaints and hazards of aging. Staying strong will help you keep up with your kids and grandkids and continue enjoying hobbies such as hiking, gardening, and golf. Aside from the obvious benefit of being physically stronger, weight training helps in other ways:

* Avoiding falls—not only by keeping you stronger, but maintaining the speed and accuracy of your body's movements

* Maintaining bone density—this is critical for avoiding osteoporosis and fractures as you age

* Keeping blood sugar under control—this has been documented in people with diabetes as well as those with only slightly impaired glucose control

Best Ways to Build Muscle

Skeletal muscle is a special type of tissue that responds to stress by becoming bigger and denser. Every time you move or speak, you're using your skeletal muscles. Walking and other moderate aerobic exercises place some demand on muscles, but not enough to encourage the development of more muscle tissue. The best way to do that is to subject your muscles to repetitive, challenging work that causes them to burn up all the sugar they're storing and demand more energy from your fat stores.

When you go through a session of weight training, the muscles you're working sustain tiny spots of damage to their fibers, called microtrauma. This is not harmful, in fact it's microtrauma that stimulates muscle hypertrophy, or growth. Aerobic exercise doesn't cause microtrauma, so doesn't contribute much stimulus for adding more muscle.

> **GOOD MOVE**
>
> Building muscles requires a healthy intake of protein, and many experts recommend getting 30 grams of protein at all three meals if you're doing weight training on a regular basis. 30 grams of protein is the amount in about 4 ounces of fish or meat.

You don't have to join a gym to get a good strength-training workout. We're going to give you some guidelines for a home workout and a gym workout, so you can choose what's most comfortable for you.

There are also many DVD and online programs for basic weight training, and we recommend that you consult one to learn good form and posture when working with weights. Check out Appendix B for some suggestions.

Building Muscle at Home Without Weights

It's possible to give your muscles a good challenge by doing calisthenics alone. One benefit to this type of exercise is that you can do it anywhere, any time, because you're just using gravity and your body's weight to create resistance.

Try this sequence of exercises for a good workout. You can add the core work described in Chapter 13 for a well-rounded muscle blast. Aim to complete two sets of 8 to 12 repetitions of each exercise:

- **Squats:** This simple exercise works all the large muscles of your legs. An important thing to remember when doing squats is to never bend your knees past a 90-degree angle to avoid excess stress on your ligaments. Your knees should never be in front of your toes. If you've had knee problems in the past, don't do squats without consulting your doctor or a physical therapist.

- **Push ups:** This exercise works your chest, abdominal, and arm muscles. It can be done with bended knees or straight legs. Make sure you focus on keeping your abdominals tight to support your back. You can even do push ups against the wall if getting down on the floor is difficult.

Working with Weights at Home

Adding weights to the calisthenics (squats and push ups) described in the previous section is a great idea, because it enables you to focus the intensity of each exercise on specific muscle groups, so as one set of muscles becomes fatigued, you can keep working by moving to another set. Here are some basic guidelines for working with weights to build muscle and burn fat:

- Begin slowly, with light weights as your body adjusts. Most women should start with dumbbells weighing about 1–2 pounds and most men can start at about 5 pounds, depending on your current strength.

- For each exercise, start with a weight you can lift about 8 times before starting to tire, and about 12 times before you need to quit.

- As you get stronger, adjust the weights you're lifting, using the same 8 to 12 rep criterion.

- Work both your *flexors* and *extensors* for balance and flexibility.

- Whatever muscle you're working on, remember to stabilize yourself by tightening your abdominal muscles.

DEFINITION

Flexors are the muscles that bend your extremities and torso. In your upper arms, the most prominent flexors are your biceps. **Extensors** are the muscles that straighten your body. In your upper arms, your triceps muscle is the most important extensor. In the legs, it's the large quadriceps muscle you can see on the front of your thighs.

Here's a short series of exercises you can do with dumbbells at home:

1. **Dumbbell step-up:** With a dumbbell in each hand, walk up a flight of stairs or use an exercise step, stepping up and back down. As you take a step, curl the elbow on the opposite side, bringing the dumbbell to your shoulder and back down again. Alternate until each side has lifted 10 to 12 times.

2. **Tricep lift:** Stand up straight, holding a single dumbbell in both hands. Lift the dumbbell in both hands straight above your head. Bend arms back behind your head so your elbows are pointing at the ceiling. Keeping your elbows still, raise the dumbbell until your arms are almost straight, then slowly lower behind your head. Repeat 10 to 12 times.

Going to the Gym

It's possible to get a great muscle workout at home, but there can be added benefits to going to a gym. At the gym, you'll find a complete set of weights for maximal flexibility in your workout. You'll also find various types of benches you can use for back extensions, sit-ups, and leg lifts.

Most athletic clubs and gyms have personal trainers on site. They can be of great help in learning good form for your exercises and avoiding injury—they also can provide you with some great motivation!

Use free weights for strength building rather than machines, unless you've had an injury or have very little muscle strength. The reason for this is that because free weights can move in all directions, lifting them requires more stability in your core and more use of small accessory muscles that maintain balance and accuracy of movement. When you use a machine, you lose much of the demand for balance and stabilization—and a chance to build more muscle.

Sequencing Your Workout

If you prefer to do all your exercising at the same time on your workout days, that's great. You should be able to get in about 30 minutes of aerobic exercise and two sets of a variety of strength-building exercises. So how do you put it all together?

Many trainers recommend that you lift weights before you jump on the treadmill or bike or take a walk, if your primary goal is optimal muscle growth and development. The reasoning is that glycogen stores are high at the beginning of a workout, so you'll be able to work harder lifting weights, promoting muscle gain. Studies have shown, however, that doing cardio first and weights second tends to burn more calories per workout than the other way around, suggesting that this sequence is best for weight loss.

The Least You Need to Know

- Strength training helps counteract the loss of muscle often seen with aging.
- Building muscle keeps your metabolic rate high, so fewer calories are stored as fat.
- Strength training can be done with or without weights, at home or in the gym.

Getting Started

Everyone has their own unique diet and exercise style. Finding out what works for you may be a bit of trial and error, but it does take some self-evaluating. In this part we'll give you the tools you need to determine what fits best into your lifestyle and personality, primarily through a series of questions to answer. Then we'll jump right into the morning hours, because this is what most people often miss out on—eating breakfast. Here we'll tell you why breakfast is so important, give you tips on how to manage this early morning meal, and provide you with a wealth of recipes to get you started. Snacks and lunches are also included here, as they are often eaten away from home and can be easily managed, especially if you brown bag it.

Taking Stock

In This Chapter

- The importance of recording your progress
- Motivate yourself with self-monitoring
- Analyze your lifestyle: diet, exercise, and stress
- Direct measures of your stress-related risks

Before you start on any big project, it's important to know where you are and where you intend to go. There are a few good reasons why it's important to take a realistic assessment of your body shape before you start working on changing it. Behavior change experts have known for decades that the person who keeps close track of her goal progression is more likely to accomplish what she set out to do than the person who doesn't.

Getting rid of your belly fat is going to involve some changes in how you eat, move, and manage stress. You're going to be very successful if you start a journal, keeping track of what you're doing now. Keeping a journal is part of the process of self-monitoring, a proven method for making behavior changes. More about journaling is discussed in the next chapter.

It's a good idea to spend a week or so tracking your behavior before you make any changes—but if you're eager to dive in, it's not absolutely necessary. But you do need to gather some baseline information before you get started.

This chapter gives you all the tools you need to make a realistic assessment about your health, your weight, your eating habits, and your physical activity as well as any risks, if any, that your body shape may be posing to your health. Knowing this information should provide you with an extra boost of motivation to make healthy changes.

Speaking of motivation, you'll want to know where you started, because after you get going on this program, your body will change quickly. There's nothing like seeing the concrete results of your efforts on paper as well as on your body!

Assess Yourself

Before you start this program, you need to make the body measurements described in Chapter 2: body weight, BMI, waist circumference, and waist-hip ratio. You may also consider getting some of the other tests discussed at the end of this chapter. In this section, you'll have the opportunity to assess your lifestyle and habits. This information will help you figure out what changes you need to make for your best results using this program.

We suggest that you complete all three of these questionnaires now, while you're in the planning stages of your flat-belly program. They cover the three pillars of the belly fat elimination program: eating, stress management, and moving. The first questionnaire will help you determine your eating style. The second will give you an idea of how much an impact stress may be having on your life. The third is an inventory of your current level of physical activity.

Eating Style Questionnaire

This questionnaire is meant to help you determine how likely it is that the way you're eating now is putting fat into your belly. Certain foods, especially sugars, white flour, and unhealthy fats, encourage your body to store extra calories in your belly. Chapter 4 looks at how that happens, but for now, let's take a look at how belly fat–prone your diet is.

Rate each item based on how accurately each statement describes your eating behavior in your regular routine using this scale:

Definitely true:	1
Fairly accurate:	2
Fairly inaccurate:	3
Definitely not true:	4

In my day-to-day life: **Response**

1. I find it hard to resist pastries, cookies, and donuts.   _____

2. I eat a salad or a vegetable side dish with at least two meals a day.   _____

3. I eat fast food at least twice a week.   _____

4. I drink soft drinks that are sweetened with sugar or corn syrup.   _____

5. I choose white bread instead of whole-wheat bread.   _____

6. I eat fish at least three times a week.   _____

7. On most days, I eat something after 8 P.M.   _____

8. I eat pasta or noodles at least twice a week.   _____

9. I regularly put sugar or honey in my coffee or tea.   _____

10. I eat dessert after dinner at least twice a week.   _____

11. I snack on candy at least two or three times a week.   _____

12. I nibble on salty snacks when I watch TV or movies at least twice a week.   _____

13. If I drink milk or eat other dairy products, they're almost always full fat/whole milk.   _____

14. I eat a whole grain like oatmeal, quinoa, or brown rice at least three times a week.   _____

15. I put full-calorie salad dressing on all salads I eat.   _____

16. I eat beef or pork at least once every day.   _____

17. I skip breakfast most days.   _____

18. I have more than one or two snacks on most days (define a snack as anything you eat between meals).   _____

19. I eat a few nuts every day.   _____

20. I put butter on most vegetables and breads that I eat.   _____

21. I eat cheese at least twice a day.   _____

22. If I'm thirsty, I'm more likely to reach for a soda, fruit drink, or juice instead of water. _____

23. I use only canola and olive oil for cooking and dressing foods. _____

24. I eat meals away from home at least four times a week. _____

25. I eat prepared food (frozen or made from a boxed product) at least three or four times a week. _____

Scoring: For items numbered 2, 6, 14, 19, and 23, you'll need to reverse the score. That is, if you rated any of these items with a 1, change that to a 4. Change a 2 to a 3, a 3 to a 2, and a 4 to a 1. This is because these items all describe eating habits you want to cultivate, and this questionnaire is designed to give you a score for unhealthy eating.

After you've reversed the scores for the 5 items mentioned, add up all responses to get your final score. The lower your score, the more likely it is that the food choices you're making now are putting you at greater risk of carrying belly fat. Don't use your score as a way to stress yourself out—take it for what it is—information. Rest assured right from the start, this lean belly program will go a long way to making your diet healthy.

You can assess your current diet with the following guidelines—if your score is …

25 or lower: You're eating a pretty standard American diet—lots of meat, salt, sweeteners, and empty calories. You're probably not getting enough fiber, fruits and vegetables, and essential nutrients from the foods you're eating. You may find the first few days on this program challenging, because you'll be making significant changes in the way you eat.

But don't worry—you'll probably have fewer blood sugar swings, fewer cravings, and more satisfaction from what you're eating after only 4 or 5 days on the program. In addition, you'll probably experience a dramatic change in your energy levels and overall well-being right from the start.

25 to 50: Your diet, while not completely unhealthy, could be improved. On my plan, you'll certainly be increasing your intake of healthy foods while cutting back on things that aren't good for you. You'll feel more energized and satisfied with the foods you're eating after only a few days on this program.

50 to 75: Looks like you're already making pretty good choices when it's time to eat. There's definitely room for improvement, though, because all of the items on this questionnaire (except the reverse scored ones, of course) should be "definitely not true" of your everyday eating habits to protect you from building up belly fat.

You may find the dietary changes in this program less challenging than others will, but you'll still notice a shift in your energy levels and overall satisfaction with what you're eating every day while your waistline shrinks.

75 to 100: Good for you—you're choosing mostly healthy foods and avoiding the biggest belly fat traps. If you're overweight or carrying belly fat, it's possible that you're eating more than you need, or you're not timing your meals and activities in such a way as to maximize your metabolic rate. Also, stress and inadequate physical activity can also lead to belly fat in even the healthiest eaters.

WHAT'S NEW

Liver fat is a hot topic in obesity research these days, because it appears that it's an even more dangerous setup for heart disease than belly fat—but the two seem to appear together, and often as a result of a diet that's too high in sugars, especially fructose.

Physical Activity Questionnaires

This questionnaire is designed to help you assess not only your formal exercise routine (if you have one) but your overall level of physical activity. Attaining and keeping a flat belly is not just about 30 minutes or so that you'll spend every day exercising. It's probably more a matter of how you spend the other 23½ hours every day.

Let's start by documenting your exercise habits.

First, let's look at your level of aerobic exercise, which benefits your cardiovascular health, endurance, and stress levels. Give yourself one point for each time per week you perform the following activities:

_____ Walk at a moderate to brisk pace for at least 30 minutes

_____ Jog or run for at least 15 minutes

_____ Ride your bike at a moderate pace for at least 30 minutes

_____ Work out on a cardio machine (treadmill, elliptical, rowing machine, stair climber, etc.) at moderate intensity (3 to 5 on a scale of 1 to 10) for at least 30 minutes

_____ Work out on a cardio machine (treadmill, elliptical, rowing machine, stair climber, etc.) at vigorous intensity (6 to 8 on a scale of 1 to 10) for at least 20 minutes

_____ Dance or engage in an aerobics class for at least 20 minutes

Scoring: Add up the points for each activity to get your overall weekly activity score. If your score is …

0 to 5: You aren't getting the minimal amount of aerobic activity that most experts recommend for avoiding heart disease, obesity, and diabetes. Being sedentary is a major risk factor for belly fat as well. As discussed in Chapter 12, daily physical activity is absolutely essential for skeletal muscle cycling of blood sugar and keeping your blood lipid profile healthy. You'll find lots of ways to go from sedentary to active in this book.

5 to 10: You're doing well—achieving at least the minimal amount of formal cardio exercise needed to minimize disease risk and keep your weight under control. If you're exercising only at low or moderate intensity, you may find that you'll lose belly fat faster if you continue exercising for the same amount of time and up the intensity. If most of your cardio is at a higher intensity, you'll probably benefit from the interval training and longer, less intense workouts described in Part 5.

10 or higher: Fantastic! You're moving your body regularly and supporting healthy skeletal tissue metabolism. If you're still struggling with your weight or belly fat with this amount of exercise, it's probably going to be very helpful to take a look at other types of exercise described in Part 5—and your eating habits and stress levels.

Now, let's take a look at your overall physical activity lifestyle. This questionnaire is meant to give you an idea of what that activity level is now, as well as inform you of several ways you can increase it. In general, the more you move around, the better able you will be to avoid belly fat buildup.

Using the following scale, rate each item based on how accurately each statement describes your behavior during a typical week:

Definitely true: 1
Fairly accurate: 2
Fairly inaccurate: 3
Definitely not true: 4

In my day-to-day life: **Response**

1. I always try to find the nearest parking spot
   when running errands.   _____

2. I spend at least 6 hours a day sitting down
   (at work and at home).   _____

3. I spend at least an hour or two every week doing
   some kind of strenuous work around home or at my job.   _____

4. When given a choice between sitting down or standing,
   I almost always choose to sit down.   _____

5. I almost never take the stairs when there's an escalator
   or elevator available.   _____

6. I commute to and from work on foot, by bike, or by
   public transportation.   _____

7. After dinner on most nights, I am usually
   watching television, reading, or at my computer.   _____

To calculate your score, first reverse your responses (0 = 4, 1 = 3, 2 = 2, 3 = 1, 4 = 0) to items 2 and 6. Then add up the values for all items to get your overall score. If your score is …

0 to 10: You're missing out on many easy, painless ways to keep your metabolism fired up and your skeletal muscles actively helping to keep your blood sugar at a healthy level. You'll lose your belly a lot faster if you adopt the habits and activities mentioned in this questionnaire.

11 to 20: You're moving around, but you could definitely be moving more. Your belly will shrink faster if you look for more ways to keep moving and avoid long periods of time spent sitting down.

21 or higher: Great! You have a lifestyle that includes a good amount of everyday physical exertion. Keep it up, and remember that every opportunity you take to move is another step toward losing that fat.

The Perceived Stress Scale

This questionnaire was developed by Dr. Sheldon Cohen in the early 1900s and has been used in hundreds of studies of stress and its effects on health. It covers several aspects of chronic stress and the thoughts and feelings that go along with it. It focuses on perceived stress rather than life events for the simple reason that stress is not about what happens to you, but about how you perceive it.

WHAT'S NEW

It's long been known that people who report feeling frequently stressed out and overwhelmed tend to get migraines and colds more often. Recently, research has uncovered a strong association between perceived stress and waist circumference in both overweight and lean people. The increase in belly fat is due to the consistently higher levels of cortisol found in the blood of people who feel high levels of stress.

These questions ask you about your feelings, thoughts, and activities during the last month, including today. In each case, write down the number that corresponds with how often you felt or thought a certain way:

0 = Never
1 = Almost never
2 = Sometimes
3 = Fairly often
4 = Very often

1. In the last month, how often have you been upset because of something that happened unexpectedly?   _____

2. In the last month, how often have you felt that you were unable to control important things in your life?   _____

3. In the last month, how often have you felt nervous and "stressed"?   _____

4. In the last month, how often have you felt confident about your ability to handle your personal problems?   _____

5. In the last month, how often have you felt that things were going your way?   _____

6. In the last month, how often have you found that you could not cope with all things you had to do?   _____

7. In the last month, how often have you been able to control irritations in your life?   _____

8. In the last month, how often have you felt that you were on top of things?   _____

9. In the last month, how often have you been angered because of events that happened out of your control?   _____

10. In the last month, how often have you felt that difficulties were piling up so high that you could not overcome them?   _____

To score the questionnaire, first reverse your responses (0 = 4, 1 = 3, 2 = 2, 3 = 1, 4 = 0) to items 4, 5, 7, and 8. Then add up all your responses. Now you can compare your score to the average scores of people in the United States, displayed in the following table.

Category	Average Score
Male	12.1
Female	13.7
Age	
18–29	14.2
30–44	13.0
45–54	12.6
55–64	11.9
65 & older	12.0

In general, a higher score corresponds with a higher likelihood that you're feeling stressed and may be experiencing some of the physical consequences of it. Studies have shown that people who score higher than average on the PSS are more likely to report symptoms of anxiety and depression and more frequent colds than those whose scores are average or below average.

If your score is relatively high, take heart. You're going to learn effective, simple ways to take control of your responses to life's hassles and obstacles.

Optional Tests to Consider

Depending on your age, health status, and physical condition, it may be advisable for you to get a checkup with your doctor and have some lab work done. In general, if you're healthy and 35 or younger, it's probably safe for you to get started without your doctor's go-ahead.

If you're between the ages of 35 and 50 and haven't had a checkup within the last year, it would be a good idea to do so. Let your doctor know about this program and what your goals are. He or she will be able to advise you of any precautions that might be necessary. If you're 50 or older, I recommend seeing your doctor before getting going on this or any other big lifestyle change.

RED FLAG

When you visit your doctor, he or she may want to do other tests unique to your situation. Conditions such as low thyroid activity (hypothyroidism) or fluctuating hormones in menopause can hinder fat loss—so be sure to discuss any and all symptoms you might be experiencing with your doctor so you are ready to lose as much of your belly as you can.

Whatever your age, you may want to consider having a few physiological indicators of stress and cardiovascular disease risk looked at before you start, so you can gauge your progress with repeat testing later. Here are a few tests that can be useful.

DIY Salivary Cortisol Test

Most drugstores now stock a take-home testing kit for assessing the amount of cortisol in your saliva. It's a simple way to get specific information about your own body's reaction to the stress in your life. There has been considerable research on the relationship between cortisol levels and belly fat, and the results are highly consistent: as cortisol goes up, so does waist circumference and many of the negative effects of belly fat. Salivary cortisol measurements, even the ones you do at home, have been shown to be a reliable indicator of the level of cortisol in your blood.

GOOD MOVE

Cortisol that's circulating in your blood is present in your saliva as well. Measuring your salivary cortisol is the easiest, least expensive way to determine your circulating cortisol levels. Most kits involve spitting saliva into test tubes, four in all, at different times of day. It's been shown that the salivary cortisol test is more reliable when four samples are collected in a single day, indicating your adrenal glands' pattern of cortisol release.

I recommend checking your salivary cortisol before you begin the flat-belly program. If it's high, you'll know you have a lot to gain by adopting one or more of the stress management techniques in this book.

Blood Pressure Monitor

Hypertension, or high *blood pressure*, is extremely common among adults in the United States, and a large number of people who have it don't know it. Government statistics show that about 29 percent of adults in the United States older than 18 have high blood pressure. The risk of hypertension goes up with age—almost 70 percent of people 60 years old or older have high blood pressure. On top of that, at least another full third of U.S. adults have prehypertension.

High blood pressure is very strongly linked to the development of heart disease and stroke. With hypertension, the heart has to work extra hard all the time, day and night, which can cause overdevelopment of the muscle tissue and abnormal heart rhythms. Another consequence of long-term high blood pressure is damage and irritation to the lining of the arteries. Any irritation to the arterial wall is a set-up for the development of atherosclerotic plaque, leading to heart attacks and stroke.

Your blood pressure should be no higher than 120/80 to be considered normal. If either number is elevated, that's evidence of hypertension. If your *systolic pressure* is between 120 and 139, and/or your *diastolic pressure* is between 80 and 89, you have prehypertension. Hypertension is defined as either systolic pressure at or higher than 140 and/or diastolic pressure at or higher than 90.

DEFINITION

Blood pressure is an indicator of how hard your heart has to work to keep your blood circulating. It's always reported as a pair of numbers separated by a forward slash. The higher number is your **systolic pressure**—the amount of force exerted by your heart when it's actively contracting. The lower number is your **diastolic pressure,** which indicates the amount of pressure remaining in your arteries when your heart is resting between beats.

I recommend that you invest in a blood pressure monitor, especially if you're 40 years or older, or you have a family member with high blood pressure. Because hypertension usually has no symptoms, screening is the best way to catch it early and take quick action to prevent it from becoming a real risk to your health. Also, stress, whether it's acute or chronic, is strongly associated with blood pressure elevations that may be transient or stable. As you work through the program in this book, chances are you'll see your average blood pressure getting lower.

Tests to Ask Your Doctor About

Depending on your level of risk for cardiovascular disease, your doctor may suggest you have your blood lipids, sugar, and inflammation markers such as C-Reactive Protein (CRP) measured. These tests are frequently part of the typical annual checkup for most people older than 40, and they're a good indication of how your diet, activity level, and stress are affecting you.

CRP is a molecule made and released by the liver in response to inflammation in any part of your body, such as the gums. High levels of CRP are strongly linked to an increased risk of heart attacks and strokes. The normal range of CRP is less than 1 mg/L. Levels between 1 and 3 mg/L are associated with average risk, and levels higher than 3 mg/L indicate a high risk of inflammation-associated disease.

People who engage in lifestyle changes such as the one in this book tend to see dramatic, beneficial changes in their blood chemistry. These changes include lower levels of LDL and total cholesterol, lower CRP levels, and elevations in HDL. Fasting blood sugar levels tend to decrease, as do blood markers of chronic inflammation.

The Least You Need to Know

- Tracking your progress is a great way to keep up your motivation.
- You can benefit more from this program if you assess your stress levels, diet, and physical activity before you start.
- It's now possible to directly measure your cortisol levels with a simple salivary test that gives you a good indication of how much stress is affecting your body.
- If you're older or concerned about other conditions, be sure and ask your doctor about other tests to monitor blood sugar and C-Reactive Protein.

Starting the Day Right

In This Chapter

- The importance of breakfast
- Sensational smoothies to maximize energy
- Quick egg scrambles to get you going
- Parfaits, pancakes, and prunes to do a belly good

It's often said that breakfast is the most important meal of the day, and, as it turns out, there is a fair amount of evidence to back this up. Numerous studies have shown that children fare better in school after a morning meal is provided and adults who consistently eat breakfast are more productive at work than those who don't. Overall, breakfast provides your body and brain with balanced blood sugar regulation, weight control through proper metabolism, and improved cognitive function. Yet despite all these positive attributes many people continuously pass over this morning meal.

This chapter not only gives you a reason to eat breakfast—getting rid of belly fat—it also gives you painless ways to prepare it, with nearly a dozen easy breakfast recipes. For those days when you're too busy to cook, there are also a bevy of delicious, nutritious smoothies to kick you into gear, and finally a recipe for ginger water to keep you hydrated throughout the day. So get ready to rev up your morning and begin making your belly fat disappear with these morning tips and recipes.

Why Eat First Thing in the Morning?

You know that breakfast is essential for refueling your body and keeping your mind active and alert, but what happens when you don't eat it? Skipping breakfast can interfere with fat loss, and when hunger kicks in, it tends to trigger eating too much to compensate. Also, the all-night fast can produce a famine response in your body, which will send you running for a quick blood sugar boost in the form of simple sugars and refined flour.

It's important to eat a breakfast high in protein because it takes longer to digest and helps keep your appetite satisfied until late morning. Also, eating protein for breakfast helps to maintain stable blood sugar levels and prevent the rush of insulin, which typically occurs immediately after a breakfast high in simple sugars, and the resultant drop, which follows a few hours later.

Ginger Water Every Morning

When losing weight, toxins, previously stored in body fat, are released. The release of these toxins may cause symptoms, such as headaches, fatigue, joint pain, achy muscles, and many others. Consider toxins if unexplained aches and pains occur when on a weight-loss diet, and protect yourself by helping the body release these toxins as efficiently as possible. While you're losing fat, it's a good idea to support your body's need to clear out previously stored toxins as they're released.

Ginger is a well-known detoxifying plant as well as a good support for digestion. Before you eat or drink anything each day, start with a glass of ginger water. This will rev up your digestive system and give a boost to the detox processes your body is going through. Here's how to make it:

1. Peel and very thinly slice a 1–2 inch segment of fresh ginger root.

2. Place the slice of ginger root in a glass container.

3. Pour a quart of near-to-boiling water over the ginger root and allow it to steep for 30 minutes.

4. Strain the liquid and discard the ginger. Store your ginger water in the refrigerator.

First thing each morning, pour yourself 8 ounces of ginger water and add the juice from a wedge of lemon. This will increase stomach acid production, preparing your body for food. You can also add a tiny pinch of cayenne pepper if you like a little spice. Cayenne is known for its ability to stimulate your metabolism, so it's great for fat loss. All in all, this little drink packs a healthy punch and it's a refreshing way to get going each morning.

 GOOD MOVE

To keep fresh ginger, store in a paper bag in the refrigerator for several weeks. If you want to keep longer, try grating it, then tightly wrapping in plastic wrap and store in freezer. This way it will keep for several months.

Have one or two 8 ounce glasses in the morning, and have another in the mid-afternoon if you're feeling a dip in your energy level. Because this drink is a bit stimulating, it's best to keep it a morning and afternoon refreshment, and have soothing herbal teas in the evening.

For Busy Mornings: The Flat Belly Smoothie

Smoothies are an easy way to maximize nutrition when time is tight. They're also a great choice on more leisurely mornings. That is, they're a great choice as long as they include the following basic elements:

- A good source of fiber
- Some protein to satisfy hunger
- High levels of vitamins and minerals
- A good source of antioxidants
- A good source of omega-3 fatty acids

One of our favorite smoothies, one you can drink almost every morning, is simple, fast, and delicious:

1. Toss a couple tablespoons of flax seeds in a blender and grind at the highest speed.

2. Add ¼ cup frozen blueberries, a scoop of protein powder or other good protein source (see chart on next page), and a scoop of a green food supplement. Green food supplements contain whole foods freeze-dried into a powder. You can find a list of brands we recommend in Appendix B.

3. Add a cup of water or, if you want something creamier, a cup of fat-free plain Greek yogurt, and blend it well.

4. If you want to add more liquid, consider water or almond milk. It's delicious and filling and gives you a huge head start on meeting each day's nutritional needs.

We recommend that you start playing around with ingredients to find your personal favorite. Here are some tips for choosing ingredients:

- Substitute frozen fruits (such as berries), which are available any time of the year, when fresh fruits are unavailable.

- High-quality protein powders can be included, but are not necessary as milk, yogurt, and tofu provide ample amounts of protein. Greek yogurt is especially high in protein.

- Vegetables are a tasty addition, and should be included liberally. From a flavor standpoint, good choices include carrots, mashed pumpkin or yams, and steamed green beans. From a nutritional standpoint, there's no reason to avoid what you like to eat.

- Fiber comes from any number of sources as seeds, fruits, and vegetables are all good options.

Use the following chart as a quick reference. Choose one or two items from each category, blend, and enjoy!

Protein Sources	Fiber Sources	Omega-3 Sources
Nonfat cow's milk	Oatmeal (cooked)	Flax seeds
Nonfat Greek yogurt	Berries	Almond butter
Lowfat soft tofu	Vegetables	Walnut halves

Quick and Easy Breakfast Recipes

Fruit Nut Parfait

This breakfast can be prepared in minutes and can even be made to go. Any fruit or nut will work in any combination—just choose your favorites. Besides being colorful and delicious, this breakfast is rich in antioxidants from the fruit, and omega-3 fatty acids and fiber from the nuts.

Yield:	Serving size:	Prep time:	Cook time:
2 cups	2 cups	5 minutes	None
Each serving has:			
370 calories	20 g fat	27 g carbohydrates	
7 g fiber	26 g protein	99 mg sodium	

½ cup each of 2 different fresh fruits, in season (raspberry and cantaloupe or honeydew, or apple and pears, or pomegranate seeds)

1 cup plain, nonfat or low-fat Greek yogurt

¼ cup roasted unsalted nuts (choose one: walnuts, pecans, almonds, pistachios, hazelnuts, or peanuts), coarsely chopped

1. If using whole fruit like cantaloupe, pears, or apples peel, core, and seed them. Dice into ½-inch pieces. If using pomegranates, cut in quarters and seed by hand. Then rinse the seeds in water.

2. In parfait glass place ½ cup yogurt, top with ½ cup fruit and ⅛ cup nuts. Repeat for second layer, ending with nuts.

3. Serve immediately or hold in refrigerator until ready to serve.

WHAT'S NEW

Yogurt is a type of fermented milk that originated in Turkey more than a thousand years ago. True yogurt contains "probiotics," or good bacteria, that can help promote a healthy digestive track and even boost your immune system.

Cottage Cheese and Melon

What can be more simple and refreshing than cottage cheese and melon? The tart, salty taste of the cottage cheese is a perfect complement to the sweet, smooth richness of the melon. This is a perfect meal for breakfast or an anytime snack.

Yield:	Serving size:	Prep time:	Cook time:
2½ cups	2½ cups	5 minutes	None

Each serving has:			
240 calories	6 g fat	35 g carbohydrates	
3 g fiber	16 g protein	325 mg sodium	

2 cups cantaloupe or honeydew melon	¼ cup low-fat plain Greek yogurt
¼ cup low-fat cottage cheese	¼ tsp. ground cinnamon
	1 TB. roasted, unsalted pumpkin seeds

1. Cut melon away from outer rind and remove seeds. Dice into 1-inch cubes.

2. In a medium bowl mix cottage cheese, yogurt, and cinnamon together until well blended.

3. Place melon in a serving bowl, and top with cottage cheese–yogurt mixture and pumpkin seeds.

WHAT'S NEW

Although the terms "muskmelon" and "cantaloupe" are often used interchangeably, they are not exactly the same. Muskmelon actually refers to a category and also includes honeydew, casaba, Crenshaw, galia, and other melons. Cantaloupe is an excellent source of vitamins A and C and a good source of potassium, fiber, B_6, folate, and B_3. Any of these melons can be substituted in this recipe.

Tropical Smoothie

Pineapple and papaya give this smoothie a tropical flair while yogurt and tahini make it smooth and creamy, giving it a nutty taste. Banana adds sweetness without added sugar.

Yield:	Serving size:	Prep time:	Cook time:
16 ounces	8 ounces	10 minutes	None

Each serving has:		
376 calories	15 g fat	48 g carbohydrates
5 g fiber	13 g protein	97 mg sodium

1 small papaya (about 1 cup)	1 sliced, frozen ripe banana
3 TB. tahini (sesame seed paste) or peanut butter	1 cup plain, low-fat or fat-free yogurt
	1 cup pineapple juice

1. Peel papaya, cut in half, and remove seeds. Coarsely chop.

2. Place papaya in a blender. Add tahini or peanut butter, banana, yogurt, and pineapple juice.

3. Blend until smooth, and serve immediately.

GOOD MOVE

The science behind making a nutritious, balanced smoothie is based on including each of the following: fiber (found in fruits, vegetables, and ground seeds), omega-3 fatty acids (found in nut butters, ground seeds, or oils), protein (found in dairy, soy, nuts, and spirulina), and vitamins and minerals (from fruits, vegetables, and nuts). The possibilities are endless.

Wilted Chard and Egg

Not only is this dish a great nutritional combination of protein and dark leafy green vegetables, but the beautiful color contrast and amazing textures make it a feast for the eyes as well as the taste buds. Leaving the egg yolk runny makes a nice sauce for the chard.

Yield:	Serving size:	Prep time:	Cook time:
1 cup	1 cup	3 minutes	7 minutes

Each serving has:		
151 calories	12 g fat	4 g carbohydrates
1 g fiber	8 g protein	230 mg sodium

1½ tsp. olive oil	2 cups Swiss chard, chopped
1 clove garlic, minced	1 egg
¼ tsp. chili powder, optional	Sea salt and ground black pepper

1. Add 1 teaspoon olive oil to small saucepan and bring to medium-high heat.

2. Add garlic and chili powder (if using) and cook 1 minute or until garlic starts to turn golden.

3. Place chard in pan and gently stir until just wilted, 3 minutes. This will cook down quickly. Transfer chard to plate.

4. Reduce heat to low and add additional ½ teaspoon oil to pan.

5. Crack egg into pan and lightly dust with salt and pepper. Let cook until white is cooked and yolk is runny.

6. Carefully flip egg and cook an additional 30 seconds.

7. Place egg on top of greens and break yolk, letting it run into greens.

GOOD MOVE

Cholesterol is not as bad as was once thought. Consequently, high-cholesterol foods such as eggs are no longer demonized and even encouraged in a healthy diet. In fact, research shows most healthy adults can enjoy an egg or two a day without any problem.

Pesto Scramble

In this Italian-style breakfast, eggs complement the pungent flavors of garlic and basil. Serve with a piece of crispy whole-wheat toast brushed with olive oil.

Yield:	Serving size:	Prep time:	Cook time:
1 egg mixture	1 egg mixture	5 minutes	5 minutes
Each serving has:			
245 calories	12.18 g fat	8 g carbohydrates	
2 g fiber	15 g protein	332 mg sodium	

½ tsp. olive oil

½ medium zucchini, ½-inch diced

2 eggs

1 TB. prepared pesto

3 cherry tomatoes, sliced in half

1. In small sauté pan heat olive oil over medium-high heat, then add zucchini and cook for about 5 or 6 minutes until zucchini becomes soft and begins to brown.

2. Whisk eggs in a small bowl with pesto. Pour over zucchini and cook over medium heat for 1 to 2 minutes, stirring gently. Cook until eggs are set.

3. Place scramble on a plate with tomatoes and serve immediately.

GOOD MOVE

The ideal egg is one that comes from a hen raised outdoors (often on pasture), eating a variety of green plants and insects, usually supplemented with a grain-based diet. Eggs from chickens who forage are nutritionally better than eggs from chickens who don't, but if you can't find grass-fed hens buy eggs from chickens fed seeds containing omega-3 fatty acids. This healthier feed produces eggs higher in omega-3 fatty acids.

Breakfast Burrito

Beans make an excellent breakfast food because they're high in fiber and protein, and keep blood sugar levels stabilized. In this burrito, beans are topped with egg, avocado, salsa, and cheese to create a multitude of flavors.

Yield:	Serving size:	Prep time:	Cook time:
1½ cups	1½ cups	5 minutes	5 minutes

Each serving has:			
300 calories	16 g fat	28 g carbohydrates	
8 g fiber	13 g protein	242 mg sodium	

¼ cup cooked beans, black or pinto, drained and rinsed

1 small corn tortilla

1 tsp. olive oil

1 egg

2 TB. salsa, fresh or low-sodium jarred

¼ avocado (about 3 TB.)

1 TB. shredded sharp cheddar, optional

1. Warm beans in a small saucepan over medium heat.

2. Heat frying pan to medium and dry heat tortilla until soft, 1 minute on each side.

3. Place tortilla on plate and top with beans.

4. Add oil to pan and crack egg into oil.

5. Cook egg until white is translucent. Gently flip egg and cook for an additional 30 seconds.

6. Place egg on top of beans. Add salsa, avocado, and cheese (if using). Roll tortilla up and serve.

WHAT'S NEW

Eggs for breakfast can be part of a smart weight-loss strategy. A study from the Pennington Biomedical Research Center showed that participants who ate two eggs for breakfast lost 65 percent more weight than participants in the same study who ate a bagel for breakfast, even though the bagel and the eggs contained an equal number of calories. The egg-eaters also lost 34 percent more belly fat and felt more energetic than the participants who ate bagels.

Recipes for Leisurely Mornings

Oatmeal Parfait

This breakfast parfait couldn't be simpler. Instead of yogurt we layer fresh fruit between creamy oatmeal, then top with a drizzle of maple syrup for a sweet topping. If you want to add some crunch, try adding a sprinkle of almonds or walnuts, too.

Yield:	Serving size:	Prep time:	Cook time:
3 ½ cups	1 ¾ cups	10 minutes	20 minutes

Each serving has:			
236 calories	3 g fat	49 g carbohydrates	
7 g fiber	7 g protein	147 mg sodium	

½ cup *steel-cut oats*, dry	1 cup fresh or frozen and thawed strawberries, sliced
1½ cups water	1½ cups fresh or frozen and thawed blueberries
⅛ tsp. sea salt	2 tsp. pure maple syrup

1. Place oats in a medium saucepan with water and salt.

2. Bring to a boil, reduce to a simmer, and cook 15 to 20 minutes, stirring occasionally.

3. In a large bowl layer half of the oatmeal, then strawberries, then rest of oatmeal, and top with blueberries. Drizzle with maple syrup. To serve, divide in half.

DEFINITION

Steel-cut oats are whole oat kernels (known as oat groats) that have been cut in small pieces by a steel blade. Rolled oats or old-fashioned oats are whole oat kernels that are steamed, flattened by rollers, and dried into flakes; quick-cooking oats are simply rolled oats that are flatter and thinner, making them cook more quickly; instant oats are the same as quick-cooking oats but they are cut in pieces and flavoring ingredients are usually added.

Curried Vegetable Scramble

Here carrots, asparagus, and green onion are cooked until crisp but tender, then blended with a creamy mixture of curried eggs. Spinach is added in at the last minute for more color, but you can use any vegetables you have on hand. For harder vegetables, like potatoes, cook them first.

Yield:	Serving size:	Prep time:	Cook time:
2 cups	1 cup	5 minutes	10 minutes

Each serving has:		
146 calories	10.8 g fat	4.2 g carbohydrates
1.2 g fiber	7.2 g protein	369.9 mg sodium

1 TB. olive oil	¼ cup fresh spinach
¼ cup green onion, chopped	2 eggs
¼ cup carrot, grated	½ tsp. *curry powder*
¼ cup asparagus, small chopped	¼ tsp. sea salt
1 garlic clove, minced	

1. Place oil in pan and heat over medium.

2. Add onion, carrot, asparagus, and garlic, and stir-fry for 3 to 5 minutes, adding spinach during the last minute.

3. Beat eggs in small bowl, adding curry powder and salt.

4. Add eggs to vegetables in pan and cook for 3 minutes, stirring occasionally until eggs become firm.

DEFINITION

Curry powder is a blend of spices usually including cumin, coriander, red chilies, mustard, and fenugreek. The mixture varies in strength and can be purchased mild or hot. Indian cooks usually make their own versions, but here in America it's easy to buy premade curry.

Cottage Cheese Pancakes with Fresh Fruit

These adorable mini pancakes make a great Saturday morning treat. Surprisingly, they contain no white flour or sugar, just puréed cottage cheese, eggs, and a dash of cornmeal. High in protein, they're a snap to make when you don't want to bother making traditional pancakes.

Yield:	Serving size:	Prep time:	Cook time:
24 pancakes	6 pancakes	5 minutes	20 minutes

Each serving has:			
191 calories	11 g fat	10 g carbohydrates	
1 g fiber	13 g protein	277 mg sodium	

1 cup low-fat or fat-free cottage cheese	2 TB. cornmeal
3 eggs	2 TB. olive oil
	1 cup fresh fruit, any kind

1. Place cottage cheese, eggs, cornmeal, and oil in blender and blend until smooth.

2. Pour batter (about 1 tablespoon batter per pancake) onto oiled frying pan over medium heat and cook for a few minutes on each side.

3. Serve with fresh fruit on the side. Strawberries, blueberries, and raspberries are all nice choices.

RED FLAG

Because most people who eat breakfast tend to eat high-carb cereal or breads, most people don't get nearly enough protein in their breakfast meal as they should (most get less than half of what they need). To pump up protein, think about adding a hard-boiled egg, cheese, beans, or lean fish or meat to your morning meal.

Warm Prunes in Orange Sauce

These warm orange-scented prunes are wonderful on their own, or as an accompaniment to hearty oatmeal, cream of wheat, or any other hot cereal. They also make a great snack when the weather is cold. If you want more of an orange flavor, try substituting orange zest for the lemon.

Yield:	Serving size:	Prep time:	Cook time:
24 prunes	6 prunes	5 minutes	20 minutes

Each serving has:		
279 calories	5 g fat	62 g carbohydrates
5 g fiber	3 g protein	2 mg sodium

1 cup fresh squeezed orange juice	½ tsp. cinnamon
1 TB. fresh lemon juice	24 pitted prunes
1 tsp. grated or minced lemon zest	¼ cup walnuts, chopped
¼ cup honey	

1. Place orange and lemon juices in a saucepan with lemon zest, honey, and cinnamon.

2. Bring to a simmer, add prunes, remove from heat, and cover tightly for 10 minutes.

3. Remove prunes, and return saucepan to heat.

4. Simmer liquid until it reduces by half and coats the back of a spoon.

5. Stir in walnuts and ladle sauce over prunes.

GOOD MOVE

Although prunes are considered a high-sugar fruit, they don't bump up blood sugar levels. That's because they're so high in fiber (10 to 12 prunes contain about 7 grams of fiber), which reduces their absorption rate. They're also a good source of potassium, vitamin K, and copper, and contain a wealth of antioxidants.

Taking It with You

In This Chapter

- Staying on track means planning ahead
- Keeping snacks and water always on hand
- Naturally nutritious nibbles
- Packing it up

Most people don't have the luxury of staying at home all day, close to the kitchen with a stockpile of healthy, nutritious foods easily at hands reach. Most of us have to go out and run errands, work outside the home, and have social lives. Being on this belly fat weight-loss program shouldn't mean that you can't be active and participate in all the things you like to do.

Check out the tips and recipes included in this chapter. They're fun, easy-to-make, and many are portable enough to stash in the car for a quick pick-me-up.

Always Plan Ahead

Snacks are an important part of any weight-loss program because they keep your metabolism humming along and they help you curb hunger between meals. Although some research shows that people who snack regularly tend to weigh more than people who don't snack, the same research also shows that most of these snacks consist of sugary drinks; candy; and salty, crunchy foods such as potato chips. A major problem with this type of snacking is that these foods trigger insulin release, which overtaxes your pancreas and can lead to a blood sugar crash, making you even more likely to snack again or eat more at your next meal.

As you work toward your lean, flat belly, you'll be supplementing your meals with healthy, delicious, and satisfying snacks. The best way to keep yourself on track is to make sure that every time you eat, you eat something satisfying and high in nutritional value.

If you don't think planning for nutritious snacks is worth it, just consider what some of the documented benefits of healthy snacking are:

- Higher metabolic rate

- Reduced tendency to overeat at mealtime

- Improved digestion of smaller quantities of food

- Reduced hunger and cravings

- Re-acclimating your stomach to smaller volumes of food

Make it part of your evening routine to look at the day ahead and strategize your eating plan based on where you're going and what you're going to be doing. A good idea is to log your plan in your flat-belly journal. If the next morning is going to be rushed, plan to have a smoothie or one of the quick breakfast suggestions in this book. You can even get your snacks and lunch ready for the next day and store them in the fridge overnight. This will cut down on any rushing around and last-minute preparations you need to do in the morning.

Your Water Bottle

Another important element in your portable flat-belly lifestyle is your water bottle. Taking water with you everywhere you go is a great strategy for keeping your belly from feeling too empty and for avoiding dehydration. Losing fat also means losing stored up toxins and flushing out extra fuel that you don't need, so keep your water bottle close at hand all day long.

GOOD MOVE

To know if you're drinking enough water, keep an eye on your urine—if it's a light shade of yellow you're doing well. If it's darker or has a strong smell, you need to drink more.

We recommend that you buy for yourself two or three nice 24-ounce water bottles. Having more than one means that if you leave one at work or in your car, you'll always have one at hand to fill before you leave home. Your water bottle should be made of BPA-free plastic or aluminum. Currently, there is some controversy around the safety of reusing the plastic bottles that water comes in, so I suggest avoiding that until more evidence comes in.

WHAT'S NEW

In a recent weight-loss study people who drank 16 ounces of water 20 minutes before each meal lost nearly 5 pounds more than nondrinkers after a 3-month period. So, drink up!

The perfect thing to put in your water bottle is, of course, water. Alternatively, you can take diluted ginger water with you. Simply pour 4 ounces of ginger water into your bottle, and fill the rest with plain water. Another option is a half and half mixture of green tea and water. If you drink coffee in the morning, limit the amount of green tea you drink per day to 12 ounces. It's a good idea to shoot for finishing off at least two full bottles of liquid a day. This will ensure that you stay well hydrated.

GOOD MOVE

Many people mistake thirst for hunger, so before you look for something to eat, grab a drink of water first. It may be all you need.

Good Ideas for Packing

To maximize your options for snacks and lunches that go where you go, consider buying an insulated lunchbox. This way, you can take salads and other healthful foods that are best kept cold with you. Most insulated lunch boxes come with a gel pack that stays cold all day after you freeze it. It's a good idea to buy a couple extras to keep on hand in the freezer so you always have a cold one.

You should also have several small- to medium-size portable, plastic food containers with tight-fitting lids. Another option is to wrap food in plastic or aluminum foil. Aside from your lunchbox, you can make sure you're never without a bite to eat by always keeping some nuts and an apple or pear in your purse or briefcase. Dried fruit is a good traveling option. Keep in mind, however that both dried fruit and nuts are concentrated sources of calories, so don't overdo it. All you need is a handful (about 1 ounce) of either (nuts or fruit) to keep you going. To prevent you from overeating, portion out amounts in a small container or plastic baggie beforehand, this way you know just how much to eat.

Snack Recipes

Guacamole

Avocado is chock-full of good-for-you fats. Try this classy rendition of guacamole with fresh vegetables cut into sticks, egg dishes, or rice crackers. It's also great for adding richness to bean dishes.

Yield:	Serving size:	Prep time:	Cook time:
1⅓ cups	⅓ cup	10 minutes	None

Each serving has:			
168 calories	15 g fat	11 g carbohydrates	
7 g fiber	2 g protein	153 mg sodium	

2 medium, ripe avocados

3 TB. onion, finely chopped

1 garlic clove, minced

½ fresh jalapeño pepper, seeded and finely chopped

1 TB. fresh cilantro, finely chopped

¼ tsp. sea salt

3 TB. lime juice

1. Halve avocados lengthwise, removing pits.

2. Scoop soft insides into a bowl, mashing with the back side of a fork.

3. Add onion, garlic, jalapeño, and cilantro.

4. Gently stir, adding salt and lime to taste. Serve at room temperature.

GOOD MOVE

Homemade dips with ingredients such as avocado or beans make nutrient-rich snacks, but remember that what you are dipping matters. Stay away from processed foods such as potato or corn chips and instead go for vegetables such as carrot and celery sticks, or red bell peppers. They contain few calories and fat, and are loaded with fiber and antioxidants.

Salmon Salad Served on Cucumber

This refreshing, crisp dish is light and satisfying. It's also high in omega-3 fatty acids. The rich salmon mixture contrasts nicely with the fresh, clean taste of the cucumber.

Yield:	Serving size:	Prep time:	Cook time:
20 rounds	5 rounds	10 minutes	None

Each serving has:		
120 calories	3 g fat	3 g carbohydrates
1 g fiber	18 g protein	121 mg sodium

1 TB. lemon juice

⅓ cup low-fat plain Greek yogurt

1 cup cooked salmon, flaked

1 clove garlic, crushed

1 TB. capers

1 TB. fresh dill, finely chopped

Pinch sea salt

Pinch ground black pepper

1 cucumber, peeled and sliced into 20 rounds

1. In medium bowl, mix lemon juice, yogurt, and salmon.

2. Add garlic, capers, dill, salt, and pepper.

3. Place cucumber rounds on platter and top each slice with 1 heaping tablespoon salmon salad. Serve each person five cucumber-salmon slices.

RED FLAG

There are challenges involved in maintaining a social life while dieting. Party food is not typically selected with weight loss in mind. To keep on track eat a healthful, filling meal *before* going out, preventing temptation, and eliminating hunger as a stumbling block to making sensible eating decisions.

Sprouted Almonds

Slightly salty and crisp, these almonds are a guilt-free pleasure. Sprouting them is easy and adds to the nutritional value.

Yield:	Serving size:	Prep time:	Cook time:
4 cups	¼ cup	24 hours	12 hours

Each serving has:			
210 calories	18 g fat	7 g carbohydrates	
4 g fiber	8 g protein	446 mg sodium	

4 cups raw organic almonds, not pasteurized

1 TB. sea salt

Warm filtered water

1. Place almonds and salt in bowl and cover with warm water, at least an inch over nuts.

2. Let sit overnight or for at least 10 to 12 hours. Almonds will take up water and swell, and you may see small white tips protruding from the narrow end of the nuts.

3. Drain water from nuts.

4. Store in refrigerator in a tightly closed container. Almonds will remain fresh for 3 to 4 days.

GOOD MOVE

Nuts are an ideal snack food because they're high in protein and fill you up (with good fats). They also contain lots of hard-to-get vitamins and minerals such as vitamin E, copper, selenium, and magnesium. Current legislation requires all domestically grown almonds to be pasteurized before sale, so until the law is overturned (almond growers are fighting it) only imported raw organic almonds can be sprouted.

Red Ants on a Log

Here's our adult version of this sweet, crunchy children's classic snack. To up the nutritional value we've used sunflower seed butter in place of the peanut butter and dried cranberries instead of raisins.

Yield:	Serving size:	Prep time:	Cook time:
12 sticks	3 sticks	5 minutes	None

Each serving has:		
115 calories	8 g fat	10 g carbohydrates
1 g fiber	3 g protein	32 mg sodium

4 celery sticks, cut into thirds

¼ cup sunflower seed butter

3 TB. dried cranberries

1. Scoop sunflower seed butter into celery sections.

2. Place cranberries about ¼-inch apart along celery tops. Serve at room temperature.

WHAT'S NEW

Celery can help lower blood pressure. Research shows that eating two sticks of celery a day can lower systolic pressure by 10 points. Scientists suspect it works by decreasing stress hormones and relaxing blood vessels. Celery also acts as a diuretic, assisting in the release of excess, retained water.

Hummus with Vegetables

High in fiber and protein, this Middle Eastern dip will give you the energy to get through the day. A great accompaniment to vegetables, on crackers, or with pita.

Yield:	Serving size:	Prep time:	Cook time:
2 cups	⅓ cup	12 hours	2 hours
Each serving has:			
191 calories	10 g fat	21 g carbohydrates	
4 g fiber	6 g protein	436 mg sodium	

½ lb. dried chickpeas, or 2 cups canned chickpeas, drained and rinsed

1 quart water

½ tsp. sea salt

3 garlic cloves

6 TB. lemon juice

½ tsp. cumin

3 TB. tahini

2 TB. olive oil

An assortment of fresh vegetables, cut into sticks

1. If using dried chickpeas, soak overnight in quart of water.

2. Drain water from peas, place peas in saucepan with fresh quart of water.

3. Bring to a boil, reduce to a simmer, cover, and cook 2 hours or until tender.

4. Drain peas then purée in food processor, while adding salt, garlic, lemon juice, cumin, and tahini.

5. Place hummus in bowl, ladle olive oil on top, and serve with vegetables (carrots, celery, and peppers are good choices).

RED FLAG

Don't let too much time go between meals. Research on satiety shows that if you wait too long (5 hours or more) you could end up eating more than if you ate several low-calorie high-fiber snacks every three to four hours.

Popcorn with Nutritional Yeast

Popcorn is a great high-fiber snack. Here, nutritional yeast gives popcorn an unexpected buttery satisfaction without the butter while delivering a good dose of B vitamins.

Yield:	Serving size:	Prep time:	Cook time:
16 cups	2 cups	5 minutes	10 minutes

Each serving has:		
110 calories	6 g fat	13 g carbohydrates
3 g fiber	3 g protein	147 mg sodium

3 TB. olive oil

½ cup popcorn kernels

½ tsp. sea salt

¼ tsp. ground black pepper

2 TB. nutritional yeast

1. Place oil in large, heavy 8-quart saucepot. Add popcorn kernels and shake, covering all sides of kernels with oil.

2. Heat pan to medium-high and cover tightly. Gently shake pan every few minutes until corn begins to pop.

3. When popping slows down to one every 2 seconds, remove from heat. Promptly remove popcorn from pan and pour into a bowl.

4. Season with salt, pepper, and nutritional yeast.

GOOD MOVE

Nutritional yeast is a fungus grown on molasses. At the end of its growth, it is pasteurized to kill the yeast. Nutritional yeast is high in minerals, B vitamins, and 18 amino acids, making it a complete protein. It is an especially valuable addition to a vegetarian's diet. Nutritional yeast is sold in stores as a powder or in flake form. It has a mild nutty or cheesy flavor and is good as a cheese substitute or on popcorn.

Apple Slices with Seed Butter

This quick snack is sure to please young and old alike. The lemon juice adds flavor and keeps the apples from turning brown.

Yield:	Serving size:	Prep time:	Cook time:
1 cup	½ cup	5 minutes	None

Each serving has:			
258 calories	15 g fat	29 g carbohydrates	
3 g fiber	7 g protein	165 mg sodium	

2 apples, cored and sliced

2 TB. lemon juice

¼ cup sunflower seed butter

1. Squeeze lemon juice over apple slices.

2. Serve with sunflower seed butter on the side for dipping.

GOOD MOVE

As soon as apples are cut, the oxygen in the air reacts with the enzymes in the fruit to turn them brown. To prevent this browning, dip apples in lemon juice or orange juice immediately. Acid stops the browning. If you want to prepare ahead of time you can also keep apples submerged in a bowl of cold water.

Trail Mix

This is a good on-the-go snack, perfect for hiking or a quick dose of protein to keep energy levels up. We love the combination of nuts, sweet fruit, and chocolate chips, but you can create any combination of seeds, nuts, and dried fruit. Adding the chocolate is optional.

Yield:	Serving size:	Prep time:	Cook time:
3 cups	¼ cup	5 minutes	None

Each serving has:		
178 calories	12 g fat	16 g carbohydrates
3 g fiber	4 g protein	2 mg sodium

1 cup cashews

1 cup almonds

1 cup dried cranberries

¼ cup chocolate or carob chips

1. Mix cashews, almonds, cranberries, and chocolate or carob chips together in an airtight container.

RED FLAG

Research shows that Americans often underestimate how many calories they consume each day by as much as 25 percent, mostly because they don't pay attention to recommended serving sizes on nutrition information labels. Many prepackaged foods contain multiple servings, even if they appear to be designed for one. Always read labels first to find out.

Flat Belly Lunches

In This Chapter

- High-protein lunches to keep your metabolic fires burning
- Super salads with grains, beans, and veggies
- Hearty soups to make at home

You did a good job eating a breakfast rich in fiber and protein. You avoided sugary breakfast treats and your blood sugar has thanked you for it. In fact, you have not craved extra caffeine or a sugary snack mid-morning as a "pick-me-up." Now it is lunchtime and you want to maintain good energy and avoid blood sugar crashes in the afternoon. What should you do?

The best way to keep metabolism high and avoid that notorious afternoon crash is to eat a meal with a healthy source of protein, balanced with some complex carbohydrates and a small amount of healthy fats. To help illustrate this, think of building and maintaining a fire. Carbohydrates are like paper or kindling—they burn quickly and brightly, but cannot maintain a healthy fire alone. Just as good steady energy cannot be maintained with carbohydrates alone.

Protein burns like branches. It provides steady energy that burns for an extended period of time. A small amount of fat translates into the log, and just as you cannot start a fire with one huge log, all calories should not come from fat sources. The best approach to build a steady fire is by incorporating the correct ratio of kindling, smaller branches, and larger logs, just as a healthy diet contains an appropriate proportion of carbohydrates, protein, and fat. To help us figure out these amounts, the current Dietary Guidelines recommend we get 10–35 percent of our calories from protein, 20–35 percent of our calories from fat, and 45–65 percent of our calories from carbohydrates.

These recipes contain just the right amount of each nutrient to burn long and slow, keeping your energy up until the next meal. Enjoy them as they are or use them as a model to build upon and create your own lunchtime meals.

Asian Quinoa Bowl

Sweet pears and savory edamame are tossed with quinoa in an Asian-style dressing. Ideal when the weather is hot or when you just want something light to eat—nutty, sweet, and savory.

Yield:	Serving size:	Prep time:	Cook time:
2 cups	1 cup	10 minutes	None

Each serving has:		
316 calories	15 g fat	38 g carbohydrates
8 g fiber	9 g protein	87 mg sodium

1 cup cooked quinoa

½ cup cooked *edamame*

1 small pear, peeled, cored, and small diced

2 TB. chopped green onions

2 TB. Asian Salad Dressing (recipe following)

¼ cup avocado, small diced

½ tsp. sesame seeds

1. In a bowl combine quinoa, edamame, pear, and green onion.

2. Drizzle with Asian Salad Dressing, gently toss together, and top with avocado and sesame seeds. Divide between two plates and serve.

DEFINITION

Edamame is the Japanese term for boiled and salted young soybeans. Soybeans are light green and round in shape (they look similar to lima beans), with a mild, sweet taste. They are usually sold frozen in a dark green, fuzzy pod. To cook edamame, just boil them in salted water, pods and all, for a few minutes.

Asian Salad Dressing

This dressing makes more than you'll need, but that's okay, simply seal it in an airtight container and put it in the refrigerator for use later on salads or vegetables. It will keep in the refrigerator for several weeks.

Yield:	Serving size:	Prep time:	Cook time:
About 1¼ cups	1 tablespoon	5 minutes	None
Each serving has:			
80 calories	8 g fat	1 g carbohydrates	
0 g fiber	0 g protein	76 mg sodium	

3 cloves garlic, crushed

2 TB. minced fresh ginger root

1 tsp. prepared Dijon-style mustard

2 tsp. honey

Juice of 1 lemon

2 TB. rice vinegar

2 TB. low-sodium tamari

½ cup olive oil

¼ cup sesame oil

1. In a food processor or with a wire whisk, combine garlic, ginger, mustard, honey, lemon, rice vinegar, and tamari.

2. Slowly drizzle olive and sesame seed oil into food processor (or if using a whisk, pour in slowly).

3. Remove mixture from processor and store in a sealed container in the refrigerator. Will keep for several weeks.

Black Bean Salad

Beans are high in fiber and protein. Here, they are perfectly matched with corn, lime juice, and cilantro. Spice up this filling salad with the addition of some hot sauce or cayenne.

Yield:	Serving size:	Prep time:	Cook time:
4 cups	1 cup	10 minutes	None

Each serving has:		
267 calories	10 g fat	38 g carbohydrates
10 g fiber	11 g protein	108 mg sodium

½ cup red onion, minced

2 cloves garlic, minced

2 cups cooked black beans

1 cup corn

½ cup red bell pepper, diced

¼ cup fresh cilantro, chopped

2 TB. olive oil

3 TB. fresh lime juice

Sea salt and ground black pepper, to taste

2 TB. roasted, unsalted pumpkin seeds, coarsely chopped

8 cherry tomatoes, quartered

1. In a medium bowl, place onion, garlic, beans, corn, pepper, and cilantro and toss together to combine.

2. In a separate bowl, blend oil, lime juice, and salt and pepper to taste to make dressing.

3. Add dressing and pumpkin seeds to corn, bean, and pepper mixture, and gently stir in tomatoes. Serve chilled.

GOOD MOVE

Pumpkin seeds are an excellent source of zinc, fiber, magnesium, and iron. They are especially beneficial for men, providing some protection against prostate cancer and benign prostatic hyperplasia. A few tablespoons a day is all you need to reap benefits.

Pita Salad Sandwich

Because it holds up so well, pita bread makes for a great salad sandwich. In this salad, salty olives, tart vinegar, and sweet grapes offer a balance of contrasting flavors that will wake up your palate.

Yield:	Serving size:	Prep time:	Cook time:
6 pita halves	2 pita halves	5 minutes	None

Each serving has:			
292 calories	10 g fat	45 g carbohydrates	
7 g fiber	9 g protein	518 mg sodium	

1 head lettuce, preferably red leaf

½ cup red onion, thinly sliced

½ cup cucumber, thinly sliced

6 black olives, thinly sliced

1 tomato, sliced

10 red grapes, cut into halves

1½ TB. olive oil

1 TB. red wine vinegar

Ground black pepper, to taste

3 whole-wheat pita breads (6½ inches in diameter), cut in half

1. Chop lettuce and place in a large bowl.

2. To lettuce, add onion, cucumber, olives, tomato, and grapes.

3. In a separate small bowl mix oil and vinegar, drizzle over lettuce, and add pepper.

4. Cut pita bread in half, open pockets, and stuff each pita half with ½ cup salad.

WHAT'S NEW

Grapes are packed with many beneficial plant compounds, of which the most famous is resveratrol. Resveratrol is found in the skin of the grapes and has been found to be protective against cancer in lab and animal studies.

Chicken Caesar Salad

Making the *Caesar dressing* yourself is easy and rewarding, not to mention better for you. Simply blend lemon juice, olive oil, garlic, and anchovy paste. Don't worry about the anchovy paste, either—it adds a layer of flavor without being fishy.

Yield:	Serving size:	Prep time:	Cook time:
5 cups	5 cups	15 minutes	None
Each serving has:			
337 calories	21 g fat	16 g carbohydrates	
6 g fiber	25 g protein	139 mg sodium	

4 cups romaine lettuce, chopped	1 tsp. anchovy paste, optional
1 medium tomato, sliced	Sea salt
¼ cup cucumber, peeled and cubed	2 oz. cooked chicken breast, cubed
2 TB. fresh lemon juice	1 TB. roasted, unsalted pumpkin seeds
1 TB. olive oil	Freshly ground black pepper, to taste
1 clove garlic, crushed	

1. Place lettuce in a large bowl; add tomato and cucumber.

2. In a separate bowl, whisk together lemon juice, olive oil, garlic, and anchovy paste (if using). Add salt to taste.

3. Drizzle dressing over vegetables and gently toss together.

4. Top with chicken, and sprinkle with pumpkin seeds and pepper.

DEFINITION

Caesar dressing was originally created on July 4, 1924, in a busy restaurant in Tijuana, Mexico. The Chef, Caesar Cardini, was running out of food for his patrons. In desperation, he searched the kitchen for ingredients and found a head of romaine lettuce, lemons, garlic-flavored oil, eggs, Parmesan cheese, and Worcestershire sauce. That day, he tossed together a masterpiece, the Caesar salad.

Spicy Southwestern Burrito

Chili powder and cayenne give this vegetarian burrito its kick, while cabbage, salsa, and low-fat sour cream cool it down.

Yield:	Serving size:	Prep time:	Cook time:
2 burritos	1 burrito	5 minutes	15 minutes

Each serving has:			
481 calories	9 g fat	80 g carbohydrates	
27 g fiber	22 g protein	518 mg sodium	

1 tsp. olive oil	⅛ tsp. cayenne pepper
½ medium red onion, diced	1 pinch sea salt
1 large red bell pepper, diced	1 cup shredded cabbage
2 cups cooked black beans	¼ cup low-sodium salsa
1 garlic clove, crushed	2 TB. low-fat sour cream
2 tsp. chili powder	2 (8-inch) whole-wheat tortillas

1. Place oil in a frying pan and bring to medium heat.

2. Sauté onion and pepper until onion turns translucent, about 5 minutes.

3. Add beans, garlic, chili powder, cayenne, and salt, and sauté an additional 10 minutes.

4. In a small bowl toss cabbage with salsa and sour cream.

5. Warm tortillas in oven or on stovetop.

6. Place 1 cup vegetable-bean mixture in center of each tortilla. Top each with ½ cup cabbage mixture, then carefully roll each tortilla, folding in ends to form burrito.

GOOD MOVE

Beans are loaded with protein and fiber and can often be used interchangeably. If you don't like black beans try pinto, small red, or kidney beans instead. There are dozens of varieties on the market.

Stuffed Grape Leaves

Inspired from the Greek dolma, these rice and pine nut stuffed *grape leaves* make a nice light lunch when the weather is hot. Briny grape leaves contribute to their tart, lemony taste, balanced by sweet raisins in the filling.

Yield:	Serving size:	Prep time:	Cook time:
12 stuffed grape leaves	4 stuffed grape leaves	20 minutes	None

Each serving has:		
183 calories	6 g fat	32 g carbohydrates
3 g fiber	3 g protein	466 mg sodium

12 cooked grape leaves

1 TB. olive oil

1 medium yellow or white onion, finely chopped

1 cup cooked brown rice

¼ cup raisins, soaked in water for 15 minutes

⅓ cup fresh dill, chopped

¼ cup fresh parsley, chopped

1 TB. toasted pine nuts

Juice from 1 lemon

1. Rinse grape leaves and set aside to partially dry.

2. Place oil, reserving 1 teaspoon, in a saucepan and heat to medium.

3. Add onion and sauté until translucent, about 5 minutes.

4. Remove from heat and stir in rice, raisins, dill, parsley, pine nuts, and lemon juice.

5. Take each individual leaf, shiny side down, and put 2 tablespoons of rice mixture on each leaf.

6. Fold the lateral ⅓ of leaf to center and roll leaf tightly from stem.

7. Drizzle stuffed grape leaves with reserved olive oil.

DEFINITION

Grape leaves are a traditional food used in Greek, Turkish, Bulgarian, and Arab cuisine. They are most often picked fresh; stuffed with a mixture of rice, vegetables, and spices; and cooked by boiling or steaming. In the United States, fresh grape leaves are hard to find. Most often you'll find them brined in a can or jar.

Tuna Tahini Salad

Using tahini (sesame paste) instead of the more traditional mayonnaise decreases the fat content, increases protein, and gives this dish a nutty flavor. Serve with pita bread or as part of a larger salad for a bigger meal.

Yield:	Serving size:	Prep time:	Cook time:
6 cups tuna mixture plus 12 cups lettuce	1 cup tuna mixture plus 2 cups lettuce	10 minutes	None

Each serving has:		
217 calories	9 g fat	11 g carbohydrates
3 g fiber	25 g protein	402 mg sodium

2 TB. tahini	Sea salt and ground black pepper
⅓ cup plain, low-fat or nonfat Greek yogurt	3 cans tuna in water, drained and flaked
Juice from 1 lemon	½ cup yellow or white onion, finely diced
2 TB. fresh parsley	½ cup celery, finely diced
4 garlic cloves, crushed	2 TB. *capers*, chopped
½ tsp. chili powder	⅓ cup toasted pine nuts, coarsely chopped
2 tsp. cumin	12 cups chopped Romaine lettuce

1. Purée tahini, yogurt, lemon, parsley, garlic, chili powder, and cumin in a food processer. Add salt and pepper, to taste.

2. In a bowl, combine tuna, onion, celery, capers, and pine nuts.

3. Gently fold dressing into tuna and vegetables. Serve tuna mixture on top of lettuce.

DEFINITION

Capers are a common seasoning ingredient in Mediterranean cuisine. The caper is actually the young flower bud of a caper plant that is then pickled and cured in salt or a salt-vinegar solution. During the curing process, the caper releases mustard oil, which gives it a distinct, intense flavor, similar to green olives. Rutin, a potent anti-inflammatory agent, is formed in them during the curing process.

Mushroom Barley Soup

Although earthy mushrooms and high-fiber barley are the main ingredients of this hearty soup feel free to add any vegetables you have on hand for extra flavor and nutrition—celery, zucchini, and broccoli all work well.

Yield:	Serving size:	Prep time:	Cook time:
8 cups	2 cups	20 minutes	40 minutes

Each serving has:			
208 calories	6 g fat	31 g carbohydrates	
5 g fiber	11 g protein	270 mg sodium	

½ cup raw pearl barley

3 cloves garlic, chopped

1 medium yellow or white onion, chopped

1 TB. olive oil

1 carrot, peeled and chopped

2 cups crimini mushrooms, cut into quarters

½ cup port, optional

6 cups low-sodium chicken or vegetable broth

1 TB. chopped fresh parsley

1 TB. chopped fresh thyme, or 1 tsp. dried thyme

1 TB. chopped fresh oregano, or 1 tsp. dried oregano

¼ tsp. sea salt

½ tsp. ground black pepper

1. Soak barley in warm filtered water overnight. Drain.

2. In medium pot, over medium heat, sauté garlic and onion in olive oil until translucent, about 5 minutes.

3. Add carrot and mushrooms; sauté an additional 3 minutes.

4. Stir in barley and port (if using), sauté another 2 minutes.

5. Add broth, increase heat, and bring to a boil.

6. Decrease heat to medium and allow to simmer until barley and carrots are tender, about 40 minutes.

7. Add parsley, thyme, oregano, salt, and pepper in last 5 minutes and serve.

WHAT'S NEW

Unlike other grains, fiber is found throughout the barley kernel and not just in the bran. On the market today you can find hulled or hulless barley (this is the least processed and most nutritious), pearled barley (polished barley), and quick-cooking barley, which is pearl barley that has been rolled and thinly shaved so it cooks quickly. Both hulled and pearl barley take about one hour to cook.

Butternut Squash Soup

This soup is creamy, delicious, and high in beta-carotene, which gives it that bright orange color. Serve it plain or with colorful garnishes to dress it up, like seafood (crab or shrimp), avocado, fresh herbs, chopped nuts, tomato, or low-fat sour cream.

Yield:	Serving size:	Prep time:	Cook time:
6 cups	1½ cups	20 minutes	1½ hours
Each serving has:			
198 calories	8 g fat	31 g carbohydrates	
5 g fiber	6 g protein	289 mg sodium	

1 2-lb. butternut squash

2 TB. olive oil

½ medium yellow or white onion, chopped

2 cups low-sodium chicken stock

1 tsp. fresh thyme

1 tsp. fresh oregano

½ tsp. kosher salt

¼ tsp. ground black pepper

2 TB. low-fat or nonfat plain yogurt

5 fresh sage leaves, finely chopped

1. Preheat oven to 425°F.

2. Cut squash in half lengthwise, remove seeds and pulp, and place on a baking dish face down. Fill pan with water to ¼-inch. Cover with aluminum foil and bake until tender, about 30 to 35 minutes. Let squash cool and then scoop out the meat. Set aside.

3. Heat oil in a large saucepot over medium heat. Sauté onion in oil until translucent, about 5 minutes.

4. Add squash, stock, thyme, and oregano, and bring to a boil. Lower heat to simmer. Add salt and pepper. Simmer for 10 minutes.

5. In batches, purée soup in food processor until smooth.

6. Return soup to saucepan and heat over medium heat until ready to serve. Top with yogurt and sage as a garnish.

GOOD MOVE

Like most orange foods, butternut squash is high in beta-carotene, the plant form of vitamin A. Beta-carotene keeps your eyes in tip-top shape and helps protect you from eye diseases, such as macular degeneration and cataracts, which can occur late in life. It also helps to enhance the functioning of your immune system and helps your reproductive system function properly.

Fish Tacos

Thanks to the Mexican influence, fish tacos are immensely popular in Southern California. In our version, the cabbage is combined with salsa and pineapple chunks for a sweet-spicy flavor.

Yield:	Serving size:	Prep time:	Cook time:
4 tacos	2 tacos	25 minutes	20 minutes

Each serving has:		
198 calories	2 g fat	34 g carbohydrates
5 g fiber	14 g protein	255 mg sodium

4 oz. white fish, cod or tilapia

1 lime, quartered

4 5-inch round corn tortillas

1 cup green cabbage, shredded

¼ cup red onion, thinly sliced

4 TB. low-sodium salsa

4 TB. crushed pineapple

1. Steam fish until firm and flaky.

2. Place fish on plate and add lime juice.

3. Warm tortillas on a dry, hot pan until soft, about 30 seconds each side.

4. Place each tortilla flat and to each add 1 ounce flaked fish, two slices onion, 1 tablespoon salsa, and 1 tablespoon pineapple.

5. Gently fold in half and serve.

WHAT'S NEW

Traditional fish tacos originated on the beaches of the Mexican Baja Peninsula, where vendors sold firm white fish, such as halibut or mahi mahi, fried in small corn tortillas with shredded cabbage laced with lime, cilantro, and a creamy sour cream dressing.

Caprese Salad

The main stars of this easy summer salad are tomatoes, basil, and fresh whole-milk mozzarella. Choose these ingredients when they're at their peak and you'll find yourself making this simple dish throughout the season.

Yield:	Serving size:	Prep time:	Cook time:
6 cups tomato-mozzarella mixture plus 4 cups mixed salad greens	1½ cups tomato-mozzarella mixture plus 1 cup mixed salad greens	10 minutes	None

Each serving has:			
193 calories	15 g fat	5 g carbohydrates	
1 g fiber	11 g protein	419 mg sodium	

2 large tomatoes (about 1 lb.), preferably heirloom, cored and diced in 1-inch cubes

6 oz. fresh mozzarella, diced into 1-inch cubes

½ cup fresh basil, loosely packed with stems removed, sliced into thin strips

2 TB. toasted pine nuts

1 TB. olive oil

1 TB. balsamic vinegar

¼ tsp. sea salt

¼ tsp. ground black pepper

4 cups mixed salad greens

1. In large bowl toss tomatoes, mozzarella, and basil together. Add pine nuts, oil, vinegar, salt, and pepper.

2. To serve, evenly divide salad greens and tomato-mozzarella mixture among four plates (about 1 cup salad greens topped with 1½ cups tomato-mozzarella mixture). Serve immediately.

GOOD MOVE

Fresh herbs and dried spices are a great way to reduce your salt intake without even noticing it. Instead of reaching for the salt shaker try experimenting with these flavorful seasoning ingredients instead: basil, dill, or oregano; curry, ginger, garam masala (a blend of spices common in India and Asian cuisines), cumin, coriander, or cinnamon; and chili powder.

Garden Wrap

This crunchy wrap filled with fresh from the garden vegetables is like a salad sandwich. Bound together with creamy high-protein hummus and a gingery-garlicky sesame seed–flavored dressing, it's ideal during the hot summer months when you want something light. Serve alongside a spinach salad and some fresh berries for a special treat.

Yield:	Serving size:	Prep time:	Cook time:
1 tortilla plus 4 cups salad	1 tortilla plus 4 cups salad	10 minutes	None

Each serving has:			
318 calories	17 g fat	36 g carbohydrates	
7 g fiber	9 g protein	505 mg sodium	

3 cups fresh raw spinach

¼ cup grated carrots

¼ cup cucumber, thinly sliced

¼ cup sprouts, broccoli or other

1 TB. Asian Salad Dressing (recipe earlier in chapter)

3 TB. hummus

1 whole-wheat tortilla

2 TB. avocado, peeled, seeded, and small diced

1. In bowl, combine spinach, carrots, cucumber, and sprouts.

2. Toss with Asian Salad Dressing to combine.

3. Spread hummus on tortilla. Top with vegetables from bowl, discarding any excess liquid.

4. Add avocado, wrap, and cut in half.

GOOD MOVE

Olive oil, a staple of the Mediterranean diet, has long been known for its health benefits. In addition to being a monounsaturated fat, it is also high in phenolic compounds, which have a protective effect against heart disease. Phenolic content is highest in virgin oils and lower in refined olive oil, so given the choice always choose extra virgin olive oil first. For simplicity's sake we used olive oil in all our recipes, but feel free to interchange that with extra virgin if you like.

Chicken Satay

Make this Thai-inspired chicken kabob the night before, then re-heat or eat cold for a smart lunch choice. It is high in protein and flavor, leaving you satisfied. Pair it with some fresh or grilled vegetables and a salad. You can also use tofu in place of chicken for a vegetarian option.

Yield:	Serving size:	Prep time:	Cook time:
1 pound	4 ounces chicken	10 minutes (plus 30 minutes to marinate)	20 minutes

Each serving has:			
233 calories	8 g fat	2 g carbohydrates	
0 g fiber	36 g protein	201 mg sodium	

1 TB. olive oil	¼ tsp. ground cumin
1 TB. light coconut milk	1 lb. boneless, skinless chicken breast
1 tsp. fish sauce	4 8-inch skewers, soaked in water for at least 2 hours
1 tsp. curry powder	
½ tsp. ground turmeric	½ cucumber, thinly sliced
1 clove garlic, crushed	

1. In a medium bowl mix together oil, coconut milk, fish sauce, curry powder, turmeric, garlic, and cumin.

2. Cut chicken into 1-inch strips.

3. Add chicken to marinade. Cover and refrigerate for 30 minutes. You can also do this step the night before.

4. Preheat oven to 425°F.

5. Thread chicken onto skewers lengthwise. Place chicken in baking dish and cook for 15 minutes. Serve with cucumber slices.

RED FLAG

Commercially sold sauces and salad dressings are typically high in sugar, often containing high fructose corn syrup, salt, and sometimes fat, derailing most people's good intentions to eat healthy. They may also contain artificial food colorings and unhealthy preservatives. Luckily, making your own sauces and dressings is easy and inexpensive. Experiment with different vinegars and herbs for healthy and delicious alternatives.

Lean Belly Plan

Losing belly fat is all about controlling your calories—balancing calories in versus calories out. Because the majority of us eat most of our calories late in the day, this part is devoted to eating in the evening hours. This includes a variety of delicious dinner meals, side dishes, and salads and desserts that you'll want to make over and over again. In conclusion we'll review the Lean Belly Plan Diet pattern and give you menu plans so you can easily adapt this way of eating to your everyday life. The result will be a slim, trim belly for life and a healthy, happy, and fit body and mind.

Time for Dinner

In This Chapter

- Quick fix dinners for when time is short
- Suppers to satisfy you all night long
- Sensational seafood meals to slim your belly

Eating meals away from home can lead to overeating and choosing unhealthy foods. Unfortunately, the old-fashioned family dinner time appears to be fading from our usual customs. More and more families pick up food on the fly, go out to eat, or grab convenience foods to eat at the end of a busy day. In fact, a recent study found that Americans spend about 40 percent of their food budget on meals outside the home, and the average restaurant meal has about 60 percent more calories than a meal made at home.

In this hectic world, many people feel that making dinner after a long day sounds like a chore. But, it doesn't have to be that way. If you plan ahead, you can get a lot of prep work and even some cooking done on the weekends. Among the recipes for dinner in this chapter, you'll find good ideas for both busy and leisurely evenings. In a pinch, you can always resort to a simple protein-veggie-grain combo and call it a day. Here are some examples:

- Leftover salmon or chicken on top of some rice or quinoa you cooked extra with a salad.

- Two scrambled eggs with a couple handfuls of veggies you keep in the fridge. Add a corn or whole-wheat tortilla.

• A can of tuna mixed with 2 tablespoons of low-fat yogurt; throw in some of your prepped veggies and pile it all on an *Ezekiel bread* or corn tortilla and heat in a toaster oven.

DEFINITION

Ezekiel bread is a type of sprouted grain bread you can usually find in your grocer's organic freezer section, or in health-food stores and specialty stores like Whole Foods or Wegman's. Because it contains legumes as well as grains, Ezekiel bread is higher in protein and vitamins and minerals than regular bread. It is also low in sodium.

The idea is to get a good 3- to 4-ounce serving of protein, balanced with some vegetable and grain sides. This way, you'll maximize your sense of fullness and get a good balance of nutrients.

You'll also notice that these recipes are heavy on seafood. Fish and shellfish are an excellent source of protein in the diet, and fatty fish are especially high in beneficial omega-3 fatty acids. (For more about omega-3s, see Chapter 5.) Dietary guidelines recommend we eat 2 to 3 servings of seafood a week, and some nutritionists suggest even higher amounts of 4 to 5 portions of seafood a week. When it comes to keeping your belly slim and trim, stick with the higher recommendations.

GOOD MOVE

Mercury is a heavy metal that is released in the air and water when fossil fuels are burned. Ingesting too much can harm our brains and nervous systems, particularly in young children and pregnant women. Mercury levels found in fish depend on the type of fish, size, age, and where it lives. Larger, older fish tend to have the highest levels. High mercury fish to avoid include: king mackerel, marlin, orange roughy, shark, swordfish, tilefish, bigeye, and ahi tuna.

Many people shy away from cooking fish at home, but with these recipes you don't have to. They're fast, easy, fool-safe, and delicious. After you've tried a few they'll become go-to recipes you can count on any day of the week.

Tandoori Chicken

Traditional Indian spices complement chicken breasts in this classic dish. Serve with a heaping side of any vegetable in season and brown basmati rice to complete the meal.

Yield: 1½ pounds	Serving size: 6 ounces	Prep time: 10 minutes (plus 1 hour to marinate)	Cook time: 25 minutes

Each serving has:		
303 calories	10 g fat	8 g carbohydrates
1 g fiber	43 g protein	445 mg sodium

2 TB. olive oil	1 cup plain, low-fat or nonfat Greek yogurt
1 tsp. ground coriander	2 TB. lemon juice
1 tsp. cumin	4 garlic cloves, minced
1 tsp. turmeric	2 TB. minced fresh ginger
1 tsp. cayenne	½ tsp. sea salt
1 TB. garam masala	1½ lb. whole boneless, skinless chicken breasts
1 TB. sweet paprika	

1. Heat oil in a saucepan over medium heat; add coriander, cumin, turmeric, cayenne, garam masala, and sweet paprika and cook until fragrant. Let cool completely.

2. In a medium bowl, whisk yogurt, lemon juice, garlic, ginger, and salt together. Add toasted spices.

3. Cut 1-inch slashes into chicken and coat in marinade. Cover and chill for at least one hour.

4. Preheat oven to a high broil.

5. Place chicken in the oven and cook each side for a few minutes, until browned.

6. Lower oven heat to 325°F and finish cooking chicken until juices run clear, about 20 minutes.

GOOD MOVE

Yogurt makes an excellent marinade for meats because it is mildly acidic (too much acid toughens meat) and contains calcium, which activates enzymes that break down protein and tenderize the meat. The more tender the meat, the shorter the cooking time.

Slow-Cooked Chicken

It takes only a few minutes of prep time to produce this juicy, tender, flavorful chicken with melt-in-your-mouth vegetables. The slow cooker does all the work. To lower the fat content of this dish, remove the skin before you eat.

Yield:	Serving size:	Prep time:	Cook time:
1 chicken	¼ chicken	10 minutes	6–8 hours

Each serving has:			
434 calories	22 g fat	21 g carbohydrates	
3 g fiber	35 g protein	637 mg sodium	

1 3-lb. whole chicken, cut into quarters

2 large carrots, peeled and cut into 1-inch pieces

2 large turnips, peeled and cut into 1-inch pieces

1 small yellow or white sweet onion, quartered

8 cloves garlic, crushed

3 TB. low-sodium soy sauce

2 TB. molasses

½ cup apple cider vinegar

1. Place chicken in a Crock-Pot with carrots and turnips.

2. In a small bowl, mix onion, garlic, soy sauce, molasses, and vinegar together. Pour over chicken.

3. Cook on low for 6 to 8 hours.

WHAT'S NEW

The first slow cooker was introduced in the 1960s and was known as a "bean cooker" or "bean pot," as canned, pre-cooked beans were not widely available then. Redesigned and renamed the Crock-Pot in the mid 1970s, it was a big success. By 1981 sales reached $30 million, as this was the perfect way for working women to get a good home cooked meal on the table.

Lemon Caper Chicken

Chicken breast gets the Mediterranean treatment with earthy capers and tart lemon. Pair it with sautéed greens and whole-wheat couscous for a delicious and colorful meal.

Yield:	Serving size:	Prep time:	Cook time:
1½ pounds chicken breast	6 ounces	20 minutes	30 minutes

Each serving has:			
382 calories	13 g fat	24 g carbohydrates	
4 g fiber	43 g protein	593 mg sodium	

4 boneless, skinless chicken breast filets (6 oz. each)

½ cup cornmeal

¼ tsp. sea salt

¼ tsp. ground black pepper

3 TB. olive oil

2 cloves garlic, crushed

1 large leek, cut into 1-inch rounds up to fibrous green part

½ cup dry sherry

1 cup low-sodium chicken stock or broth

2 lemons, one squeezed, one sliced thinly

2 TB. capers

2 TB. fresh Italian parsley, finely chopped

1. Place chicken breasts between parchment paper and pound lightly with a meat mallet or rolling pin until ¼-inch thick.

2. Combine cornmeal, salt, and pepper in a small dish, bowl, or plate.

3. Heat 1 tablespoon oil in a sauté pan over medium-high heat.

4. Add garlic and leek and sauté until soft and translucent. Remove from pan and set aside.

5. Heat remaining 2 tablespoons of olive oil in the sauté pan.

6. Dredge both sides of chicken breasts in cornmeal mixture, shake off any excess cornmeal.

7. Place chicken in pan over medium-high heat and sauté about 2 minutes on each side, or until golden brown. Remove and cover while you make the sauce.

8. To the same pan, add sherry and cook for about a minute, scraping up sides until slightly thickened, then add stock or broth, lemon juice, and capers to the pan. Mix in leek-garlic mixture and heat.

9. Return chicken to the pan and bring it to a boil, then down to a simmer and cook for about 10 minutes. The liquid should be reduced. Add chopped parsley just at the end of cooking.

10. Garnish with sliced lemons. Serve immediately.

GOOD MOVE

Choose white chicken meat over dark when you can. One serving (3½ ounces) of white meat contains 3.6 grams of fat and 1 gram saturated fat, while the same size serving of dark meat contains 11 grams of fat, of which 3 grams are saturated. White meat is also higher in protein than dark meat.

Polenta with Red Sauce

Polenta is a common staple in northern Italian cuisine, but instead of butter these hearty squares are topped with a rich tomato sauce. If you want a bit more texture try adding sautéed Portobello mushrooms, zucchini, or peppers and onions. It's a great alternative to pasta.

Yield:	Serving size:	Prep time:	Cook time:
4 cups	1 cup	5 minutes	1½ hours

Each serving has:			
329 calories	8 g fat	60 g carbohydrates	
4 g fiber	6 g protein	607 mg sodium	

2 TB. olive oil

2 cups *polenta* (yellow cornmeal)

8 cups water

4 cloves garlic, chopped

1 tsp. sea salt

2 cups canned or homemade low-sodium tomato sauce

Grated Parmesan cheese (optional)

Fresh basil, finely chopped (optional)

1. Preheat oven to 350°F.

2. Grease a shallow 4-quart baking dish. In this dish combine oil, polenta, water, garlic, and salt. Stir with a fork.

3. Bake uncovered for 1 hour and 20 minutes.

4. Stir polenta with a fork and then bake for an additional 10 minutes.

5. To serve, spoon polenta onto a plate, top with tomato sauce and sprinkle with Parmesan cheese and basil, if using.

DEFINITION

Polenta is an Italian word for ground cornmeal boiled in water. In this country it refers to both the dish and the cornmeal that it is made from. It can be soft and creamy or firm and dry (able to slice and fry), depending on what you are using it for. In northern Italy, polenta is prepared in many different ways and is more popular than pasta.

Tomato Basil Soup

Make this soup when tomatoes are at their peak and basil is plentiful. Sweet, creamy, and rich-tasting, this basil-scented soup can be served hot or cold. It tastes like summer in a bowl.

Yield:	Serving size:	Prep time:	Cook time:
8 cups	2 cups	10 minutes	30 minutes

Each serving has:			
125 calories	4 g fat	21 g carbohydrates	
6 g fiber	4 g protein	592 mg sodium	

1 TB. olive oil

1 medium yellow or white onion, finely chopped

4 garlic cloves, minced

8 large tomatoes, cored, seeded, and cubed

1 TB. no-salt added tomato paste

2½ cups low-sodium vegetable broth

1 tsp. ground black pepper

1 tsp. kosher salt

1 TB. finely chopped fresh basil or ½ tsp. dried basil

1. Heat oil in a medium saucepan. Add onion and sauté until soft and translucent, about 3 to 5 minutes.

2. Add garlic and sauté until fragrant, about another minute.

3. Add tomatoes, tomato paste, broth, pepper, and salt.

4. Bring to a boil, reduce to a simmer, and then cook for 10 minutes and stir in fresh basil. Purée in blender for 2 minutes until smooth (be careful, it's hot). Serve immediately.

GOOD MOVE

Tomatoes are high in lycopene, an antioxidant that is used to treat and prevent prostate cancer. In the skin, lycopene protects against sun-mediated oxidative damage that can lead to wrinkles, sun spots, and cancer. Other foods that have lycopene include watermelon, pink grapefruit, papaya, guava, and apricots.

Sautéed Shrimp and Fennel

Fennel has an anise-like flavor that mellows when it's cooked. In this Mediterranean-style recipe, shrimp is briefly tossed with fennel, tomatoes, and capers. Serve on a bed of brown rice with a side of roasted Brussels sprouts.

Yield:	Serving size:	Prep time:	Cook time:
8 cups	2 cups	10 minutes	20 minutes
Each serving has:			
253 calories	7 g fat	16 g carbohydrates	
4 g fiber	33 g protein	429 mg sodium	

1 TB. olive oil

1 large fennel bulb, cored and cut into 2-inch-long strips

5 large tomatoes, diced

1 TB. chopped fresh thyme

2 TB. chopped fennel fronds (greens)

1 lb. raw medium shrimp, peeled and deveined

2 TB. capers

¼ tsp. ground black pepper

1. Heat oil in a large sauté pan over medium heat.

2. Add fennel bulb and cook, stirring occasionally, for about 6 to 8 minutes, until strips begin to brown.

3. Add tomatoes, thyme, and fennel fronds while stirring to scrape up bits on the bottom of the pan.

4. Add shrimp and cook for about 2 to 3 minutes until pink and just cooked through.

5. Stir in capers and black pepper and serve.

GOOD MOVE

There are actually two edible parts of the fennel plant—the bulb, which grows underground, and the feathery fronds on top. Both have a licorice-like flavor. Used much the same way celery is, fennel can be cooked or eaten raw. In the Mediterranean the fennel bulb is often eaten raw as an appetizer or after dinner, as it promotes digestion.

Seared Scallops

The richness of scallops is treated with a Thai-inspired sweet-spicy sauce, tinged with chili peppers and honey.

Yield:	Serving size:	Prep time:	Cook time:
1 pound	4 ounces	10 minutes	10 minutes

Each serving has:			
176 calories	7 g fat	8 g carbohydrates	
0 g fiber	19 g protein	580 mg sodium	

1 garlic clove	1½ TB. water
1 small fresh hot chili, seeded and chopped	1 TB. fresh lime juice
2½ tsp. honey	1 lb. medium sea scallops
2 TB. rice vinegar	Sea salt and ground black pepper
2 TB. *fish sauce*	1 TB. olive oil
	1 cup baby bok choy

1. Mash garlic, chili, and honey into a smooth paste.

2. In small bowl, mix paste with vinegar, fish sauce, water, and lime juice until well blended. Set aside.

3. Pat scallops dry and brush both sides with olive oil. Season with salt and pepper.

4. Brush a sauté pan with remaining oil and heat over medium-high heat. Add scallops to pan, turning over once, until seared and cooked through.

5. In the meantime, steam bok choy, about 5 minutes.

6. Arrange scallops on bok choy and drizzle with garlic-chili-fish sauce. Serve immediately.

DEFINITION

Fish sauce, or *nam bplah* in Thai, is made from salted and fermented fish and water. It is a staple in Southeast Asian cooking, and imparts a distinct aroma and flavor. High-quality fish sauce is typically made from anchovies, mackerel, and/or sardines.

Baked Salmon

In the Northwest you can find salmon prepared in a million different ways. Here it's baked with an olive oil–balsamic vinegar dressing flavored with fresh cilantro, fresh basil, and lots of garlic. This is by far one of my favorite dishes.

Yield:	Serving size:	Prep time:	Cook time:
2 pounds	About 5 ounces	10 minutes	15 minutes

Each serving has:		
253 calories	11 g fat	1 g carbohydrates
0 g fiber	35 g protein	408 mg sodium

½ cup olive oil

¼ cup balsamic vinegar

4 cloves garlic, minced

2 lb. wild salmon filets, boneless and skinless, cut in 5-ounce pieces

1 TB. fresh cilantro, finely chopped

1 TB. fresh basil, finely chopped

1 tsp. kosher salt

1. Preheat oven to 400°F.

2. Mix together oil and vinegar in a small bowl.

3. Rub garlic on salmon filets and place them in a baking dish.

4. Pour vinegar and oil mixture over salmon and then season with cilantro, basil, and salt. Let marinate for 10 minutes.

5. Remove salmon from marinade and place in roasting pan. Put in oven and bake for 15 to 20 minutes, turning once. It should flake easily with a fork, but maintain a darker pink in the middle. Serve immediately.

GOOD MOVE

Choose wild salmon over farmed when you can. While wild salmon can be found in both the Atlantic and the Pacific Oceans, it's the Pacific that has the most environmentally healthy populations. Depending on what time of year it is, the species you can expect to see are Chinook, Chum, Coho, Pink, and Sockeye.

Zesty Steak

If your family likes steak on the grill, this is one recipe you're going to love. The orange-thyme marinade gives the meat just a hint of sweetness combined with the smokiness of the grill. Try it with some grilled vegetables and a side salad.

Yield:	Serving size:	Prep time:	Cook time:
1 pound	¼ pound	30 minutes	20 minutes

Each serving has:		
222 calories	8 g fat	1 g carbohydrates
0 g fiber	34 g protein	220 mg sodium

2 TB. yellow or white onion, finely chopped

4 TB. orange juice

Zest of one orange

2 TB. fresh thyme

½ tsp. ground black pepper

¼ tsp. sea salt

4 4-ounce beef tenderloin filets or any lean steak

1. Combine onion, orange juice, zest, thyme, pepper, and salt.

2. Rub spice mix into steaks.

3. Place steaks in refrigerator for at least 30 minutes.

4. Place steaks on grill over medium heat, discard any leftover marinade, and grill steaks to desired doneness.

RED FLAG

Beware of grass-fed meat that's grain finished the last month of the animals' life. (It's usually stated on the label.) Eating grain even for this short period changes the fatty acid composition of the meat, negating any of the benefits of grass-fed meat.

Halibut with Avocado-Grapefruit Relish

This meaty, steak-like fish holds up well to the tartness of grapefruit and the creamy richness of avocado. Try it with a side of coconut rice.

Yield:	Serving size:	Prep time:	Cook time:
1 pound	6 ounces	10 minutes	10 minutes

Each serving has:			
400 calories	19 g fat	22 g carbohydrates	
5 g fiber	37 g protein	426 mg sodium	

Juice of one large grapefruit	1 tsp. honey
1 tsp. grapefruit zest	1 TB. chili powder
½ avocado, peeled, cored, and diced	1 tsp. ground black pepper
1 small shallot, minced	¼ tsp. sea salt
1 TB. fresh cilantro, chopped	2 6-ounce filets, boneless, skinless halibut
2 TB. fresh basil, chopped	1 TB. olive oil
1 tsp. apple cider vinegar	

1. Preheat oven to 400°F.

2. In a small bowl combine grapefruit juice and zest, avocado, shallot, cilantro, basil, apple cider vinegar, and honey. Set aside.

3. In a small shallow pan mix chili powder, pepper, and salt. Dredge fish in spice mixture, patting on both sides.

4. Heat oil in a sauté pan over medium-high heat. Add halibut and sear 30 seconds on each side.

5. Place fish in oven and bake 10 minutes or until flakey.

6. Serve with avocado-grapefruit relish.

GOOD MOVE

Why sea salt over table salt? Besides the inferior flavor, iodized table salt contains dextrose (a refined sugar derived from corn); synthetic iodine; and an anti-caking agent, calcium silicate. Sea salt is harvested from oceans and dried by the sun. It is a rich source of trace minerals, otherwise hard to obtain. Table salt is mined from the earth and is highly processed to remove trace minerals. Unless specified, any "salt" used in these recipes should be sea salt.

Poached Cod in Tomato-Caper Sauce

Poaching is one of the healthiest ways to cook fish, as it is a gentle method that preserves flavor without adding excess fat. Because cod is loaded with good-for-you omega-3 fatty acids, it is one of the better fish choices. A zesty sauce adds Italian accents.

Yield:	Serving size:	Prep time:	Cook time:
12 ounces	6 ounces	10 minutes	15 minutes

Each serving has:			
274 calories	13 g fat	7 g carbohydrates	
1 g fiber	32 g protein	353 mg sodium	

1 qt. water, salted	1 TB. capers, chopped
1 TB. olive oil	1½ TB. fresh thyme, chopped
1 shallot, minced	1 tsp. balsamic vinegar
1 cup cherry tomatoes, halved	¼ tsp. ground black pepper
¼ cup kalamata olives, sliced in half	12 ounces cod filet (2 6-ounce pieces)

1. Put water in a medium saucepan on stove to boil.

2. Heat olive oil in a small sauté pan over medium heat. Add shallot and cook for about 30 seconds.

3. Add tomatoes and cook until softened, about 1½ minutes. Then stir in olives and capers, cooking for 30 seconds more.

4. Stir in thyme, vinegar, and pepper. Remove from heat and set aside.

5. After water reaches boil, lower it to a very low simmer. Gently place fish in water and cook for 3 to 4 minutes on each side until done. Remove fish from water.

6. Serve fish with tomato-caper sauce drizzled over.

GOOD MOVE

Poaching is a gentle cooking method where food is cooked in liquid heated to 160°F to 180°F, which means the water barely shows signs of bubbles. Simmering occurs at a higher temp, from 185°F to 205°F, during which bubbles form on the bottom and rise to the top. Boiling is where bubbles break the surface at 212°F. The best way to poach is to bring the liquid to a boil then reduce the heat to a poaching temp before adding the food.

Chickpea and Rice Stew

Indian spices mixed with chickpeas, rice, and sweet potatoes make this a hearty, filling, vegetarian stew perfect for cool weather nights. You can switch up the vegetables depending on what you have on hand and up the heat with chili pepper if you like it hot.

Yield:	Serving size:	Prep time:	Cook time:
9 cups	1½ cups	30 minutes	1 hour

Each serving has:			
381 calories	6 g fat	68 g carbohydrates	
10 g fiber	14 g protein	380 mg sodium	

1 TB. olive oil	2 15-oz. cans chickpeas, drained and rinsed
1 medium yellow or white onion, chopped	3 cups sweet potato, peeled and small-diced
2 tsp. cumin	⅔ cup brown rice
2 tsp. coriander	¼ tsp. sea salt
½ tsp. turmeric	¼ tsp. ground black pepper
1 cup orange juice	½ cup fresh parsley, chopped
4 cups low-sodium chicken stock or broth	

1. Heat oil in a large sauté pan over medium heat; add onions and cook until soft and browned, about 10 minutes.

2. Add cumin, coriander, and turmeric, and stir for 20 seconds until toasted and fragrant.

3. Add orange juice, stock, chickpeas, sweet potatoes, rice, and salt.

4. Bring to a boil, and then reduce to a low simmer and cover.

5. Stir occasionally for about 45 minutes, until the rice is cooked and the sweet potatoes are breaking apart. Season with pepper and garnish with parsley.

GOOD MOVE

This recipe uses canned beans, but you can try your hand at dried if you'd like. Simply soak the beans overnight in water, drain, add fresh water, and cook until tender (about an hour or so).

Saffron Bulgur

Fresh herbs brighten up this whole-grain side dish, enhanced with colorful vegetables, pine nuts, and saffron, and finished off with a squeeze of fresh lemon juice. Perfect by itself as a light lunch or a side dish with grilled meat, fish, or poultry.

Yield:	Serving size:	Prep time:	Cook time:
8 cups	2 cups	10 minutes	40 minutes

Each serving has:			
213 calories	8 g fat	31 g carbohydrates	
6 g fiber	8 g protein	481 mg sodium	

1 cup *bulgur* (#2, medium grind)

2 cups low-sodium chicken stock

10 strands saffron

½ medium yellow or white onion, chopped

2 cloves garlic, minced

1 red bell pepper, chopped

1 zucchini, chopped

1 cup lightly packed fresh cilantro, finely chopped

½ cup lightly packed fresh basil, finely chopped

½ tsp. chili powder

1 tsp. ground black pepper

½ tsp. sea salt

3 TB. lemon juice

Zest of 1 lemon

¼ cup toasted pine nuts

1. In cast-iron skillet, lightly toast bulgur over medium heat for a few minutes, stirring occasionally.

2. Add stock, saffron, onion, garlic, bell pepper, and zucchini. Bring to a boil.

3. Remove from heat, cover, and let sit for 30 minutes or until tender.

4. Remove lid, stir in cilantro, basil, chili powder, black pepper, and salt. Continue to cook until any excess water has cooked off, about 5 minutes.

5. Stir in lemon juice, zest, and pine nuts. Taste and adjust seasoning for salt and pepper. Serve.

DEFINITION

Bulgur is whole wheat that is first steamed or parboiled, dried, and then crushed or ground. A staple in Middle Eastern cuisine it is available in fine (#1), medium (#2), or coarse (#3) grinds. Bulgur is high in protein and fiber, making it good for weight loss. One cup of bulgur has fewer calories, less fat, and more than twice the fiber of one cup of brown rice.

Lentil Stew

The combination of ginger and chili powder gives this spicy lentil stew a kick, while the extra vegetables make this a hearty and satisfying meal. Simple and filling, this soup is good on a cold day or when you're coming in out of the rain. It's good served over brown rice.

Yield:	Serving size:	Prep time:	Cook time:
8 cups	2 cups	10 minutes	1 hour

Each serving has:			
215 calories	7g fat	28 g carbohydrates	
6 g fiber	12 g protein	450 mg sodium	

1 TB. olive oil	2 large carrots, peeled and cut into large chunks
1 medium yellow or white onion, diced	1 zucchini, cut into large chunks
2 cloves garlic, minced	3 celery stalks, cut into large chunks
2 TB. fresh ginger, minced	4 cups low-sodium chicken or vegetable stock
½ tsp. chili powder	½ cup brown lentils
1 tsp. cayenne pepper	1 bunch fresh parsley
½ tsp. sea salt	2 sprigs fresh thyme

1. Heat olive oil in a large saucepot over medium-high heat. Add onion, garlic, ginger, chili powder, cayenne, and salt. Cook until onions are soft and translucent.

2. Add carrots, zucchini, and celery, and sauté for 5 minutes.

3. Pour in stock and lentils. Bring to a boil, and then reduce heat and simmer for 45 minutes or until lentils are tender.

4. Add parsley and thyme, and cook 5 minutes longer. Serve.

GOOD MOVE

Lentils are brimming with fiber (1 cup cooked has nearly 16 grams of fiber), making them an ideal weight-loss food. Foods high in soluble fiber satisfy hunger more quickly than other (low-fiber) foods, thus reducing appetite. They also keep you feeling full longer.

Lemony Lamb Soup with Barley

Another winter dish that is warm and filling. Adding the lemon juice and the peas in at the last minute gives this dish a bright, light flavor that complements the earthiness of the lamb and barley.

Yield:	Serving size:	Prep time:	Cook time:
8 cups	2 cups	20 minutes	1 hour

Each serving has:			
390 calories	12 g fat	39 g carbohydrates	
9 g fiber	34 g protein	259 mg sodium	

1 TB. olive oil	4 cups low-sodium chicken stock or broth
1 lb. lamb stew meat cut into cubes	½ cup pearled barley
½ medium yellow or white onion, diced	2 cups fresh-cooked or frozen thawed peas
2 medium carrots, peeled and cut into ½-inch pieces	Juice and zest of 2 lemons
2 medium stalks celery, cut into ½-inch pieces	½ tsp. ground black pepper
	½ tsp. sea salt, optional

1. Heat oil in a 4-quart pot over medium-high heat. Add lamb and brown on all sides.

2. Add onions, carrots, and celery. Sauté until lightly browned (about 5 minutes).

3. Add stock to the pot and bring to a low simmer. Do not boil!

4. Stir in barley and cook covered for 45 minutes until barley is tender.

5. Add peas, lemon juice and zest, pepper, and salt (if using), and simmer for 5 minutes.

6. Ladle into bowls and serve.

GOOD MOVE

Like all red meat, lamb is an excellent source of protein. It also supplies a healthy dose of iron, zinc, niacin, and vitamin B_{12}. To keep saturated fat in check, be sure and trim all visible fat.

Chili-Lime Shrimp and Pineapple Kabobs

Pineapple becomes smokey sweet when threaded on skewers and grilled with chili spiked shrimp, green peppers, and onion. This light lunch or supper is perfect for a backyard barbeque.

Yield:	Serving size:	Prep time:	Cook time:
10 skewers	2 skewers	10 minutes	10 minutes

Each serving has:		
338 calories	9 g fat	27 g carbohydrates
4 g fiber	38 g protein	508 mg sodium

10 12-inch skewers

2 cloves garlic, minced

½ cup fresh cilantro, chopped

1 tsp. chili powder

2 TB. olive oil

Juice and zest from 1 lime

½ tsp. sea salt

2 lb. large shrimp, peeled and deveined

2 green bell peppers, cut into 2-inch pieces

1 large yellow or white onion, cut into 2-inch pieces

4 cups fresh pineapple, cut into 2-inch pieces

1. Soak skewers in water for 30 minutes.

2. In a small bowl combine garlic, cilantro, chili powder, oil, lime juice and zest, and salt.

3. Pour marinade into a zipper lock bag with shrimp, peppers, and onion and coat well. Refrigerate for 30 minutes.

4. Alternately thread shrimp, pepper, onion, and pineapple onto skewers, sliding them down the skewer so they sit tightly together. There should be 4 pieces of each item on each skewer.

5. Grill on medium, about 4 to 5 minutes on each side, until nicely browned.

GOOD MOVE

Grilling fruit on the barbecue carmelizes sugars and concentrates flavor. It's also a great way to up your fruit intake, particularly if paired with savory dishes like meat, fish, or chicken. The best part is almost any fruit can be grilled on the barbecue, if done carefully.

Sole En Papillote

In this all-in-one meal, *sole* is steamed with fresh vegetables and herb cilantro, creating a complete packet of goodness. To change things up vary the vegetable and the herb—think zucchini and basil.

Yield:	Serving size:	Prep time:	Cook time:
4 pouches	1 pouch	10 minutes	10 minutes

Each serving has:		
143 calories	4 g fat	3 g carbohydrates
1 g fiber	22 g protein	391 mg sodium

1 TB. olive oil	1 TB. fresh cilantro, chopped
¼ fennel bulb, cut into thin strips	½ tsp. sea salt
½ leek, cut into thin strips	½ tsp. freshly ground pepper
½ red bell pepper, cut into thin strips	4 4-ounce sole filets

1. Preheat oven to 450°F.

2. Fold 4 12-inch square pieces of parchment paper in half. Starting from the folded side, cut into half-heart shapes.

3. Open up and brush the parchment hearts with olive oil.

4. Toss fennel, leek, and bell pepper with cilantro, salt, and pepper, and divide evenly among 4 parchment papers, placing vegetable mixture on one-half of parchment hearts.

5. Lay a sole filet on top of each bed of vegetables.

6. Fold parchment in half and fold edges closed to seal.

7. Cook in oven for 8 to 10 minutes, until parchment is brown.

8. Slice envelopes open and serve immediately.

DEFINITION

Sole is a very mild, delicate white fish which cooks quickly. At the store you may find Dover sole, lemon sole, or petrale sole (a Pacific flounder). Because sole can be expensive and hard to find, feel free to substitute with flounder or cod.

Walnut-Encrusted Tilapia with Blueberry Compote

Although it may sound unusual, blueberries and seafood are natural partners, as the sweet berry balances the robust flavor of the fish. A walnut crust adds crunch and richness, not to mention a bevy of vitamins and minerals.

Yield:	Serving size:	Prep time:	Cook time:
1½ pounds	6 ounces tilapia	10 minutes	8 minutes

Each serving has:		
436 calories	18 g fat	24 g carbohydrates
5 g fiber	49 g protein	394 mg sodium

1½ cups fresh blueberries	½ cup whole-wheat flour
½ tsp. ground black pepper	½ tsp. sea salt
4 sprigs thyme, leaves removed	½ cup walnuts, finely chopped
Juice and zest of ½ lemon	1½ lb. tilapia filet (4 6-oz. pieces)
1 TB. balsamic vinegar	1 TB. olive oil
½ cup low-fat milk	

1. Mash blueberries, pepper, thyme, lemon juice and zest, and vinegar in a 1½-quart pot and bring to a low boil on medium heat. Reduce to simmer for 2 minutes and remove from heat when done. Set aside.

2. Place milk in a small shallow bowl. Combine flour, salt, and walnuts in another small shallow bowl.

3. Dredge each filet first in milk then in chopped walnut-flour mixture, coating evenly on both sides by gently pressing down. Heat oil in large sauté pan over medium heat. Place filets in pan and brown for about 2 to 3 minutes on each side, until golden brown.

4. Place filets on plates and top each with about ¼ cup blueberry compote. Serve immediately.

GOOD MOVE

Walnuts are a rich source of good fats, omega-3 fatty acids, and alpha-linolenic acid (ALA), as well as vitamin E and the trace minerals copper and manganese. As part of a healthy diet walnuts can help protect against heart disease, high blood pressure, inflammation, and Type 2 diabetes.

White Bean and Pumpkin Soup

Pumpkin is the secret ingredient that transforms this white bean soup from ordinary to extraordinary. Colorful, flavorful, and full of good nutrition, it is perfectly suited for the earthy beans and fall flavors of sage and thyme.

Yield:	Serving size:	Prep time:	Cook time:
8 cups	2 cups	15 minutes	2 to 3 hours

Each serving has:			
320 calories	7 g fat	47 g carbohydrates	
15 g fiber	22 g protein	442 mg sodium	

½ lb. dried white beans	2 quarts low-sodium chicken stock or broth
3 cups water	½ lb. pumpkin, peeled and chopped
1 TB. olive oil	½ tsp. sea salt
1 small yellow or white onion, small diced	1 tsp. ground black pepper
2 cloves garlic, minced	1 TB. fresh thyme
	1 TB. fresh sage

1. Soak beans in water overnight, drain, rinse, and set aside.

2. Heat oil in a large saucepot over medium heat.

3. Add onion and garlic and sauté until soft and translucent, about 2 or 3 minutes.

4. Add beans and stock or broth to pot and bring to a boil.

5. Reduce heat and simmer covered for 2 to 3 hours. When beans are almost tender, add in pumpkin. Cook for an additional 45 minutes.

6. Add salt, pepper, thyme, and sage, and cook an additional 5 minutes.

GOOD MOVE

More than just for pie, pumpkin is a highly nutritious vegetable. Cooked similarly to squash, it's loaded with beta-carotene (the plant form of vitamin A), zeaxanthine, which is good for the eyes, and a slew of B vitamins.

Steamed Thai Mussels with Lemongrass

Lemongrass, Thai basil (a spicier cousin to Italian basil—if you can't find Thai basil, Italian basil will work), and chili peppers give these steamed mussels a Southeast Asian flair. Serve it over some brown jasmine rice and steamed broccoli for a complete and delicious meal.

Yield:	Serving size:	Prep time:	Cook time:
2 pounds mussels	½ pound mussels	5 minutes	10 minutes

Each serving has:			
269 calories	8 g fat	19 g carbohydrates	
1 g fiber	30 g protein	680 mg sodium	

2 lb. mussels

3 stalks lemongrass

2 tsp. olive oil

½-inch piece fresh ginger, smashed

4 garlic cloves, crushed

1 Thai chili pepper, seeded and finely chopped

2 cups low-sodium chicken stock or water

Juice of 1 whole lime

½ cup lightly packed Thai basil, roughly chopped

1. Wash and clean mussels. Be sure and de-beard (removing the string on the outside) them. Discard any mussels that are dead or have cracked or broken shells. Set aside.

2. Cut lemongrass into 2-inch pieces and gently mash with the back of a fork to release juices.

3. In a large saucepan, heat oil over medium heat. Add lemongrass, ginger, garlic, and chili pepper. Sauté for 1 or 2 minutes until soft and fragrant.

4. Mix in chicken stock or water, lime juice, and basil. Bring to a simmer. After liquid is simmering add in mussels, cover tightly, and simmer until mussel shells open completely, about 4 minutes. Serve immediately.

DEFINITION

Lemongrass is a perennial plant originally native to India. It has a light lemony flavor that is often paired with garlic, lime, cilantro, or chilies, and is common in Thai and Vietnamese dishes. The entire stalk is used. (Beware of woody stalks, as they are old.) You can find lemongrass at specialty Asian stores.

Salads and
Side Dishes

In This Chapter

- Eating vegetable dishes that make your mouth water
- Making super salads you can rave about
- Jumping on the whole grain train
- Making the best of beans and legumes

Eating vegetables is one thing you can always feel good about. In Chapter 6, we covered the many benefits of eating vegetables, inspiring you to find ways to add them to your diet. Unfortunately, some people are under the impression that vegetables are expensive and time consuming to eat every day. In reality, it only takes a little extra thought and effort to make sure you reap all the benefits of an ample intake of veggies every day. Plus, ounce for ounce, fresh vegetables more often than not come out cheaper compared to processed convenience foods.

Start by investing in a mini food processor—it's worth its weight in gold because it makes quick work of preparing any vegetable and clean up is easy. Next, set aside some time once or twice a week for a vegetable prep session. This will only take about 20 minutes. First, chop one or two cups each of onions, bell peppers, and celery sticks, either by hand or in your mini processor. Next, shred 2 or 3 large carrots with your cheese grater. Finally, separate the leaves from a head or two of romaine lettuce. Thoroughly wash and dry them, but leave them intact to preserve moisture. You can do this with a number of different vegetables. Store all of your prepped veggies separately in lidded containers or plastic baggies in the fridge.

This makes preparing many of the recipes in this chapter a breeze. Another tip is to make dishes ahead when you can. Some of the salads, like Festive Roasted Peppers, actually get better as they sit.

Don't think of eating vegetables as a chore. With their bright colors, vibrant flavors, and unusual textures, they are one of the easiest and fastest ways to add excitement and creativity to a meal. Explore the recipes in this chapter with an open mind—swap out vegetables, change up grains, and tailor it to what you and your family like. Be creative and soon you'll be preparing your own vegetable creations.

Tuna Cannellini Salad

This is a hearty salad, one you can throw together in a flash. You can make this with canned beans, or ones you've cooked yourself. Feel free to substitute other herbs if you don't have sage.

Yield:	Serving size:	Prep time:	Cook time:
3½ cups	1¼ cups	10 minutes	None
Each serving has:			
442 calories	16 g fat	41 g carbohydrates	
11 g fiber	35 g protein	289 mg sodium	

2 TB. olive oil

2 TB. red wine vinegar

⅓ cup red onion, finely chopped

1 garlic clove, finely minced

3 TB. fresh parsley, finely chopped

4 tsp. chopped fresh sage or
   1 tsp. dried sage leaves

1 (15-oz.) can drained and rinsed or
   1¾ cups fresh cooked cannellini
   beans (white kidney beans)

1 (6-oz.) can solid white tuna packed in
   water, drained well

½ tsp. ground black pepper

4 large iceberg lettuce leaves

1. Whisk oil and vinegar together in a medium bowl.

2. Add onion, garlic, parsley, and sage.

3. Mix in beans and tuna. Season with pepper.

4. Line a bowl or platter with the lettuce leaves and top with salad.

GOOD MOVE

Cannellini beans are the largest of the three most often used white beans. The others are great northern beans, which are smaller, with a nutty, dense flavor, and navy beans, which are the quickest to cook because of their very small size. Feel free to try any or all of these beans in this recipe for variety.

Black Bean and Corn Salad

This colorful Mexican-inspired salad can be served on a bed of shredded romaine lettuce or used as a hearty filling for wraps and tortillas. Finish it off with a drizzle of olive oil and a squeeze of more zesty lime juice.

Yield:	Serving size:	Prep time:	Cook time:
4 cups	⅔ cup	15 minutes, plus 2 hours chill time	None

Each serving has:			
100 calories	1 g fat	19 g carbohydrates	
4 g fiber	5 g protein	180 mg sodium	

1½ cups canned black beans, drained and rinsed

1 cup yellow corn

2 medium green onions, finely chopped

¾ cup red bell pepper, finely diced

1 TB. flaxseeds

1 tsp. ground cumin

Juice from 3 limes (or 6 TB. lime juice)

½ tsp. sea salt

½ tsp. ground black pepper

1. In a medium bowl mix beans, corn, onions, and bell pepper together.

2. Add flaxseeds, cumin, and lime juice. Toss lightly, and add salt and pepper.

3. Chill for 1 to 2 hours in the refrigerator, then serve. Store leftovers in a covered container in the refrigerator.

GOOD MOVE

You can reduce the sodium content of canned beans by 40 percent by rinsing beans under cold water. And don't worry, you won't wash away any of the nutrients in the beans—only the salt!

Chopped Niçoise Salad

In France this tuna-tomato–green bean salad typically includes steamed potatoes. Here we've skipped the potatoes in lieu of more vegetables but still kept the characteristic caper-mustard-lemon dressing. It's a great main dish lunch salad.

Yield:	Serving size:	Prep time:	Cook time:
12 cups	3 cups	15 minutes	None

Each serving has:		
330 calories	18 g fat	20 g carbohydrates
6 g fiber	24 g protein	615 mg sodium

2 TB. fresh lemon juice

2 TB. red wine vinegar

2 garlic cloves, finely minced

1 tsp. Dijon mustard

1 cup chopped fresh basil or 2 TB. dried

3 TB. olive oil

5 TB. plain, low-fat or nonfat Greek yogurt

1 small head green leaf or Boston lettuce, torn into bite-size pieces

3 large tomatoes, chopped into 1-inch pieces

1 green bell pepper, chopped into 1-inch pieces

1 small cucumber, chopped into ½-inch pieces

3 medium carrots, peeled and chopped into ½-inch pieces

½ lb. green beans, trimmed, steamed until slightly tender, and cut into 1-inch pieces

3 hard-boiled eggs, quartered, then each quarter cut in half

1 (6-oz.) can solid white tuna, drained, and separated into chunks

8 canned anchovy fillets, drained

8 kalamata or other brine-cured black olives, cut in half

1. Combine lemon juice, vinegar, garlic, mustard, and basil in a small bowl.

2. Use a wire whisk to mix in the olive oil and yogurt. Set aside.

3. Arrange lettuce on a large plate.

4. Arrange tomatoes, bell pepper, cucumber, carrots, green beans, and egg wedges on top of lettuce on the plate.

5. Crumble tuna chunks over vegetables. Arrange anchovies and olives on top.

6. Pour vinaigrette over the salad and lightly toss everything together. Serve immediately. (If not serving salad right away, do not add dressing. Cover and keep in refrigerator for up to 4 hours.)

Beet Salad

This simple Moroccan-inspired salad looks beautiful on the plate. Seasoned with cumin, paprika, and cinnamon it is a flavorful Middle Eastern accompaniment to grilled fish or chicken. If you want to add some crunch, top it with some walnuts.

Yield:	Serving size:	Prep time:	Cook time:
4 cups	⅔ cup	30 minutes, plus 1 hour chill time	10 minutes

Each serving has:			
88 calories	5 g fat	11 g carbohydrates	
4 g fiber	2 g protein	75 mg sodium	

2 lb. beets, cut into 1-inch cubes

½ tsp. ground cumin

½ tsp. paprika

¼ tsp. ground cinnamon

1 tsp. lemon zest

2 TB. olive oil

Juice from 1 lemon

Sea salt and ground black pepper, to taste (optional)

4 TB. chopped fresh parsley

1. Steam beets until tender, about 10 minutes. Transfer to a medium bowl.

2. To beets add cumin, paprika, cinnamon, lemon zest, oil, lemon juice, and salt and pepper, if using.

3. Cover and chill in refrigerator for at least an hour.

4. Toss in parsley just before serving.

GOOD MOVE

Beets have a wonderful rich, red color that can stain your tablecloth and napkins if you're not careful. To remove a beet juice stain, immediately place the item under cold running water and let it rinse for about 30 seconds. Then treat it with a stain prewash solution, letting that sit for 10 minutes or so. If the stain remains after rinsing away the prewash, try soaking overnight in a 50-50 mixture of oxygen-based bleach and water. Repeat this step until the stain is gone, then launder as usual.

Fennel, Pear, and Romaine Salad with Vinaigrette

Fennel has a distinct licorice-like flavor that plays well off the sweet crispness of the pear and mildness of romaine lettuce. Tossed with a lemony dressing, this winter salad is ideal when the weather is cold.

Yield:	Serving size:	Prep time:	Cook time:
4 cups	1 cup	10 minutes	None

Each serving has:			
180 calories	11 g fat	22 g carbohydrates	
7 g fiber	3 g protein	158 mg sodium	

2 TB. olive oil	½ tsp. ground black pepper
2 tsp. lemon juice	1 fennel bulb
1½ tsp. grated lemon zest	2 *pears,* Bartlett or Comice
2 tsp. fennel greens, chopped	6–8 walnuts, broken into pieces
1 TB. chopped parsley	½ head of romaine lettuce, thinly sliced
½ tsp. sea salt	

1. In a small bowl whisk oil and lemon juice together until thickened.

2. To this mixture add lemon zest, fennel greens, parsley, salt, and pepper. Set dressing aside.

3. Trim fennel bulb and thinly slice.

4. Core pears, then thinly slice lengthwise, the same size as the fennel.

5. In a large bowl, gently toss fennel, pears, walnuts, and romaine lettuce with dressing. Serve immediately.

DEFINITION

The **pear** is a cousin of the apple that originated in Central Asia. Asian pears are the oldest known cultivated pear, and are crisp and juicy like an apple, but with a taste similar to a sweet pear. The Comice pear is a round pear with an apple-like shape and a green hue tinged with a red blush; the flavor is sweet, succulent, and buttery. Bartlett pears are yellow or green with a pear-like shape. They are the juiciest pear and have a mild sweet flavor.

Cucumber Avocado Salad

The crisp, crunchy cucumber and creamy avocado are two summer fruits that complement each other beautifully in this simple Asian-inspired salad. Chili peppers give it a nice kick!

Yield:	Serving size:	Prep time:	Cook time:
3 cups	½ cup	5 minutes	None
Each serving has:			
102 calories	8 g fat	6 g carbohydrates	
2 g fiber	1 g protein	115 mg sodium	

1 large avocado, peeled and pit removed

2 cucumbers, peeled

2 TB. sesame seed oil

2 tsp. *tamari*

¼ tsp. chili flakes

2 tsp. rice vinegar

1. Chop avocado and cucumber into ½- to 1-inch cubes. Place in a medium bowl.

2. In another small bowl combine oil, tamari, chili flakes, and vinegar. Whisk thoroughly.

3. Pour dressing over cucumber and avocado and toss together gently. Serve immediately.

DEFINITION

Tamari is a Japanese variety of soy sauce that, unlike regular soy sauce, is made almost completely from soybeans and contains no wheat. Compared to regular soy sauce, tamari is thicker and richer, with a smooth flavor that many people prefer over regular soy sauce. Choose low-sodium tamari when you can.

Summer Quinoa Salad

Quinoa has a mild nutty flavor unlike any other grain, but after you try it we're sure you'll be hooked. It's also the only grain that is a complete protein, supplying a hefty amount of all the nutrients you need to stay healthy. In this recipe its nuttiness is enhanced by dry roasting it in a skillet before adding liquid. It also gives it a browner hue.

Yield:	Serving size:	Prep time:	Cook time:
4 cups	1 cup	10 minutes, plus 1 hour chill time	30 minutes

Each serving has:			
275 calories	13 g fat	33 g carbohydrates	
5 g fiber	7 g protein	261 mg sodium	

1 cup quinoa	½ tsp. ground black pepper
1¾ cups water or low-sodium chicken broth	1 bunch radishes, trimmed and diced
3 TB. olive oil	1 bunch green onions, both white and green part, chopped
2 TB. lemon juice	1 bunch parsley, chopped
½ tsp. sea salt	1 cucumber, peeled, seeded, and diced

1. Place quinoa in a saucepan over medium heat and cook, stirring constantly, for about 2 or 3 minutes until toasted. You should begin to smell a nutty flavor. Be careful not to burn.

2. Add water or broth and bring to a boil. Reduce heat to medium-low and simmer, covered, until liquid is absorbed, 10 to 15 minutes. Remove from heat and let sit, covered, about 2 minutes.

3. In a separate bowl, whisk together oil, lemon juice, salt, and pepper. Set aside.

4. Fluff quinoa with a fork. Add radish, green onion, parsley, and cucumber. Toss gently with dressing. Refrigerate for an hour and then serve.

GOOD MOVE

Quinoa is known as a superfood because it is one of only two plant foods that contain all eight essential amino acids, meaning it is a complete protein. (The other one is soybeans.) Most quinoa is already pre-rinsed and steamed, but if not, rinse the grain before you cook it to remove saponin residues, which can have a bitter taste.

Festive Roasted Peppers

These peppers make a flavorful and brightly colored side dish. You can also cut them into strips and serve on an antipasto platter. Roasting concentrates their flavor.

Yield:	Serving size:	Prep time:	Cook time:
2 cups	½ cup	15 minutes	None

Each serving has:			
129 calories	10 g fat	8 g carbohydrates	
3 g fiber	1 g protein	245 mg sodium	

2 red bell peppers	1 TB. fresh oregano or fresh basil, finely chopped
2 yellow bell peppers	½ tsp. coarse sea salt or kosher salt
2 garlic cloves, finely minced	¼ tsp. ground black pepper
3 TB. olive oil	
¼ tsp. balsamic vinegar	

1. Char peppers under the broiler, turning often until blackened all over (about 4 minutes).

2. Remove peppers from the oven and enclose in a paper bag. Let stand for 10 minutes.

3. While peppers are cooling, mix garlic, oil, vinegar, oregano or basil, salt, and pepper together in a medium bowl.

4. Peel charred skin from peppers and remove seeds.

5. Cut peppers into large slices.

6. Place peppers in bowl with olive oil mixture and toss. Season with salt and pepper.

7. Cover and chill in refrigerator for at least 3 hours before serving.

WHAT'S NEW

All peppers start out green and then eventually turn their true color—red, yellow, orange, purple, etc. Red peppers, in particular, are high in vitamin A (containing 9 times more than green peppers) and vitamin C (two-thirds more than green peppers).

Curried Brown Rice with Raisins and Pine Nuts

Raisins and pine nuts give this classic curried rice dish a sweet and savory taste that goes well with chicken or fish. For a change, switch out the pine nuts for almonds or cashews.

Yield:	Serving size:	Prep time:	Cook time:
4½ cups	¾ cup	10 minutes	1 hour

Each serving has:			
215 calories	7 g fat	36 g carbohydrates	
2 g fiber	4 g protein	211 mg sodium	

1 TB. olive oil

1 medium carrot, peeled and small diced (¼-inch)

1 small yellow or white onion, small diced (¼-inch)

¼ cup pine nuts

1 cup brown rice

2¼ cups water

1½ tsp. ground curry powder

¼ cup raisins

½ tsp. sea salt

2 TB. fresh lemon juice

1. In a large saucepan heat 2 teaspoons olive oil over medium-high heat. Add carrot and onion, and cook for about 1 or 2 minutes. Then add pine nuts. Stir until pine nuts become toasted and brown, about 3 or 4 minutes.

2. Mix in rice, stirring until rice is coated with oil, for about 1 or 2 minutes.

3. Add water, curry powder, and raisins. Bring water to a boil.

4. Cover, reduce heat to low, and simmer until rice is tender and water absorbed, about 40 minutes.

5. When rice is done fluff with fork, and sprinkle with salt and remaining 1 teaspoon olive oil mixed with lemon juice. Gently mix together. Serve immediately.

GOOD MOVE

To save time in the kitchen, cook 2 cups of raw rice for this recipe, then set the extra 3 or so cups of cooked rice aside for another day. You can mix it with cooked vegetables, beans, or greens for another meal or two later in the week.

Lentils with Swiss Chard

Earthy lentils come to life in this hearty fall dish. Swiss chard can be substituted with most any other leafy green such as spinach or kale.

Yield:	Serving size:	Prep time:	Cook time:
3 cups	½ cup	10 minutes	30 minutes

Each serving has:			
195 calories	7 g fat	24 g carbohydrates	
11 g fiber	10 g protein	126 mg sodium	

1 cup green or brown lentils, sorted and rinsed	3 cloves garlic, minced
1 bay leaf	½ tsp. ground coriander
3 TB. olive oil	1 tsp. ground cumin
1 medium yellow or white onion, chopped (¼-inch dice)	1 bunch Swiss chard, roughly chopped
	Sea salt and ground black pepper

1. Place lentils in a medium saucepan with bay leaf and enough water to cover by 3 inches.

2. Bring to a boil, then lower heat to a simmer until lentils are tender, about 25 minutes. Drain and set aside. Remove bay leaf.

3. Meanwhile, heat oil in a medium skillet over medium-high heat.

4. Add onion and sauté until golden, about 10 minutes.

5. Add garlic, coriander, and cumin, and sauté an additional minute.

6. Add chard to saucepan and cook until wilted, 1 to 2 minutes.

7. Stir lentils into chard mixture and serve. Add salt and pepper to taste.

WHAT'S NEW

Unlike other legumes, lentils need no presoaking and cook quickly in less than an hour. Do not, however, salt these legumes until after they are cooked, as salt will toughen their skin.

Spicy Sautéed Broccoli

Broccoli is a hearty vegetable that takes well to strong flavors. Here it is paired with two of my favorites, spicy garlic and hot chili flakes.

Yield:	Serving size:	Prep time:	Cook time:
2⅔ cups	⅔ cup	5 minutes	15 minutes

Each serving has:			
156 calories	10 g fat	14 g carbohydrates	
6 g fiber	5 g protein	57 mg sodium	

1 bunch broccoli, about 1–2 lb.	¼ tsp. chili flakes
3 TB. olive oil	1 lemon, cut into wedges
3 garlic cloves, minced	Sea salt and ground black pepper to taste

1. Chop broccoli into small florets, peel and chop stems.

2. Steam broccoli until tender, about 10 minutes. Drain and rinse briefly with cold water.

3. Heat oil on medium in a medium skillet. Add garlic and chili flakes, and cook until garlic begins to turn golden, about 1 minute.

4. Add broccoli to skillet and turn repeatedly until coated.

5. Season with salt and pepper, and serve with lemon wedges.

DEFINITION

Broccoli is part of the cruciferous vegetable family named after its cross-shaped flowers. Packed with powerful phytochemicals, like sulforaphane, broccoli protects against cancer, infection, inflammation, and heart disease.

Roasted Root Vegetables

Roasting *root vegetables* intensifies their sugars, giving these vegetables a sweet interior and crispy, caramelized exterior. Easy and delicious, even people who don't like vegetables will love this dish. It's perfect served with grilled fish or meat.

Yield:	Serving size:	Prep time:	Cook time:
4 servings	1 cup	5 minutes	30 minutes

Each serving has:			
164 calories	10 g fat	17 g carbohydrates	
5 g fiber	2 g protein	78 mg sodium	

3 small beets, peeled and chopped into ½- to 1-inch pieces

2 parsnips, peeled and chopped into ½- to 1-inch pieces

2 carrots, peeled and chopped into ½- to 1-inch pieces

½ yellow or white onion, chopped into ½- to 1-inch pieces

3 TB. olive oil

1 TB. balsamic vinegar

Sea salt and ground black pepper

1. Preheat oven to 400°F.

2. Toss beets, parsnips, carrots, and onion in bowl with oil, vinegar, salt, and pepper.

3. Place vegetables in a shallow pan or baking sheet and bake in oven until tender, about 20 minutes, turning after 10 minutes. Serve immediately.

DEFINITION

Root vegetables are the underground or starchy root of a vegetable plant. They contain a wealth of vitamins and minerals and store well during the winter months. Root vegetables include carrots, beets, turnips, rutabaga, parsnips, potatoes, and radishes, to name a few.

Pesto Quinoa

A delicious alternative to pasta, quinoa holds the garlic and basil of *pesto* beautifully. Plus, all of the added nutritional benefits of a whole grain make this a winning side.

Yield: 2⅔ cups	Serving size: ⅔ cup	Prep time: 10 minutes	Cook time: 20 minutes
Each serving has:			
107 calories	8 g fat	8 g carbohydrates	
3 g fiber	1 g protein	8 mg sodium	

1 large eggplant, peeled and sliced lengthwise into ½-inch slices	2 cups water
2 tsp. olive oil	¼ cup store-bought pesto
⅛ tsp. sea salt	1 cup cherry tomatoes, cut in half
1 cup quinoa	¼ cup coarsely chopped walnuts

1. Turn oven on broil. Cover a sheet pan with aluminum foil and spray with cooking spray. Place eggplant slices on foil and brush with olive oil. Sprinkle with salt.

2. Broil eggplant slices until soft and tender and slightly brown (about 5 to 10 minutes). Watch carefully so they don't burn. Remove from oven and set aside to cool.

3. Place quinoa in a medium saucepan with water, bring to a boil, cover, and reduce heat. Cook for 20 minutes or until tender.

4. While quinoa is cooking chop eggplant into ½-inch pieces.

5. When quinoa is cooked, remove lid and let cool 10 minutes.

6. Stir in pesto, cherry tomatoes, and roasted eggplant. Sprinkle with walnuts. Serve immediately.

DEFINITION

Originating from the fishing village of Liguria in Italy, where basil grows wild, **pesto** gets its name from the word *pestle,* from the mortar and pestle used to make it. Traditional recipes use just a few ingredients—basil, extra virgin olive oil, sea salt, and garlic.

Braised Cabbage

Braising cabbage results in a buttery texture and flavor. This dish is a great accompaniment to chicken, red meat, or other vegetable dishes.

Yield:	Serving size:	Prep time:	Cook time:
6 cups	1 cup	10 minutes	1 hour

Each serving has:			
125 calories	7 g fat	16 g carbohydrates	
4 g fiber	2 g protein	130 mg sodium	

1 small head green cabbage, cored and chopped into 1-inch pieces	1 medium carrot, peeled and chopped into $\frac{1}{2}$-inch pieces
$\frac{1}{2}$ yellow or white medium onion, chopped	3 TB. olive oil
	1 tsp. caraway seeds, optional
1 small eating apple, peeled, cored, and chopped	$\frac{1}{2}$ cup water
	$\frac{1}{4}$ tsp. sea salt
	$\frac{1}{2}$ tsp. ground black pepper

1. Preheat oven to 350°F.

2. Combine cabbage, onion, apple, carrot, oil, and caraway seeds (if using) in a large bowl.

3. Transfer to a 9 × 13 roasting pan. Add water and cover with foil.

4. Bake covered for 45 minutes, stirring occasionally.

5. Uncover, raise the oven temperature to 400°F and bake for 15 to 20 minutes more, until cabbage gets slightly brown on the edges. Sprinkle with salt and pepper, toss together, and serve.

GOOD MOVE

During the seventeenth and eighteenth centuries Northern European sailors carried vitamin C–rich cabbage on their ships to stave off scurvy. The high-fiber vegetable also contains significant amounts of manganese, iron, and vitamin B$_6$.

Collard Rolls

Collard greens make great wraps for anything you don't want to enclose in bread. In this dish, the carbohydrates are on the inside in the form of rice and vegetables, and ginger gives it an Asian twist.

Yield:	Serving size:	Prep time:	Cook time:
12 rolls	2 rolls	30 minutes	30 minutes

Each serving has:		
103 calories	4 g fat	8 g carbohydrates
3 g fiber	8 g protein	265 mg sodium

⅓ cup olive oil	1 large beet, peeled and grated
4 cloves garlic, minced	2 medium carrots, peeled and grated
2 tsp. grated ginger	2 cups green or red cabbage, shredded
¼ cup maple syrup	1 cup cooked brown rice or other grain
2 TB. low-sodium tamari	2 bunches collard greens (or 12 large leaves)

1. Preheat oven to 350°F.

2. Whisk oil, garlic, ginger, maple syrup, and tamari in a small bowl. Set aside.

3. In another larger separate bowl, combine shredded beets, carrots, and cabbage.

4. Pour marinade over vegetables and let sit for 30 minutes.

5. Transfer vegetables to baking dish and bake for 30 minutes, stirring once.

6. Remove vegetables from oven and stir in cooked rice or other grain.

7. Lightly blanch collard greens, and gently remove bottom half of spine, careful not to tear collard.

8. Place ¼ cup rice vegetable mixture at base of each collard leaf.

9. Carefully fold outer ¼ of leaf toward the center, and roll the leaf upward until fully rolled.

DEFINITION

Although **collard greens** are a member of the cabbage family, they look more like a dark leafy green. Boiled or simmered, they are a traditional dish in the Southeastern United States that was introduced to this country by West African slaves in colonial times.

Lemony Kale

This simple dish is made in minutes, but the flavor makes a lasting impression. Tart lemon is the perfect compliment to kale's mildly bitter taste, and the hearty greens make a great match for winter stews and soups. A pinch of chili pepper gives it a kick.

Yield:	Serving size:	Prep time:	Cook time:
2 cups	½ cup	5 minutes	5 minutes

Each serving has:			
80 calories	7 g fat	4 g carbohydrates	
1 g fiber	2 g protein	266 mg sodium	

1 bunch kale, chopped into 1-inch strips	1 TB. tamari
1 TB. lemon juice	2 TB. olive oil
	¼ tsp. chili flakes, optional

1. Steam kale for 5 minutes or until it wilts.

2. Transfer to a bowl, and add lemon juice, tamari, and oil.

3. Sprinkle on chili flakes (if using) and serve immediately.

GOOD MOVE

A cool-weather leafy green and member of the cabbage family, kale is considered one of the healthiest vegetables on the planet, thanks to super-high levels of vitamins A, C, and K; antioxidants; and sulfur-containing phytonutrients. It can be eaten raw or cooked and ranges in taste from mild to pungent and bitter tasting, depending on the variety.

The Sweet Side of Life: Desserts

In This Chapter

- Savor small-size sweets
- Let fruit satisfy your sweet tooth
- There's always a place for chocolate

Ah, dessert! When they wanted a sweet treat, people in ancient civilizations indulged in fruit or nuts rolled in honey. That was it. In fact, for most of our history, there was no such thing as ice cream, cakes, cookies, and the like.

Today, we've taken the concept of a tiny sweet to dangerous extremes. What used to be a treat is now a habit for many people. No longer is "dessert" saved for after dinner—but the plethora of candy bars and packaged pastries has encouraged us to become a nation of all-day sugar noshers. If you want to lose belly fat, you have to get a handle on your desire for sweets and learn to use them as occasional delights enjoyed in moderation.

One of the goals of this program is to help you switch off your "sweet tooth" and learn to love the wide variety of flavors available in whole, unprocessed foods. For this reason, desserts are limited to once per day and only in small amounts. The dessert recipes in this chapter shine for their use of healthy, nutritious ingredients and their small serving sizes.

Moderation Is Key

When deciding to eat dessert, serving size is key to avoiding excess calories. Because many desserts are high in fat and sugar, this is critical to prevent weight gain. Here are some ways to keep your sweet tooth in check:

- **Share desserts.** Don't order an individual dessert for yourself. A few bites are enough to satisfy without packing on calories.

- **Use fruits to satisfy cravings for sweets.** Fruits contain sugars and taste sweet, but they also contain fiber, vitamins, and minerals, adding to their healthy attributes. Fruit is also low in calories and more filling than refined sugars and flours.

- **Make desserts from scratch.** Avoid refined foods such as cane sugar and white flour. These foods are void of nutrition and actually drain your body of vitamins during the digestion process.

- **Remove sweet snacks from the house.** If there are leftovers from baking or entertaining, freeze them or, better yet, give them away to others.

- **Drink water or herbal tea with dessert.** Water increases satiety more quickly without adding any calories.

GOOD MOVE

Use the principles of mindful eating when you have dessert—slow down, savor, and really appreciate this tiny gift you're giving yourself. When this becomes a habit, you'll know you've taken charge of your tastes and desires, and you'll have a powerful tool for eliminating and preventing belly fat.

Dessert Recipes to Feel Good About

Chocolate Sesame Bars

An adaptation of the Middle Eastern dessert halva, this combination of chocolate and nuts is rich and filling.

Yield:	Serving size:	Prep time:	Cook time:
6 squares	3 squares	10 minutes	None

Each serving has:			
198 calories	14 g fat	16 g carbohydrates	
4 g fiber	6 g protein	297 mg sodium	

3 TB. sesame seeds	¼ tsp. vanilla extract
3 TB. almonds	½ tsp. ground cinnamon
1 TB. raw *cacao* powder	Pinch of sea salt
1 TB. honey	

1. Using a very clean coffee grinder, grind sesame seeds and almonds into a fine meal.

2. Transfer to a bowl, and stir in cacao powder, honey, vanilla extract, cinnamon, and sea salt.

3. Place mixture into a 3 × 3-inch tin, and press firmly into bottom of tin; or you can simply shape into 3 × 3-inch square using waxed paper.

4. Refrigerate for 2 to 3 hours until firm.

5. Cut into ½-inch squares. Place in a sealed plastic container and store in refrigerator.

DEFINITION

Cacao literally translates to "food of the gods" for its rich, intense flavor. The words cacao and cocoa are sometimes used interchangeably, but in the United States, cacao refers to the raw, unprocessed beans, and cocoa is the name used after the beans have been roasted and pulverized into a fine powder.

Fruitsicles

This is a great summer treat to take with you on an after-dinner stroll. The citrus in this recipe is bright and refreshing, but you can use other fruit flavors. Get creative.

Yield:	Serving size:	Prep time:	Cook time:
2 fruitsicles	1 fruitsicle	10 minutes	None

Each serving has:			
161 calories	4 g fat	28 g carbohydrates	
0 g fiber	4 g protein	71 mg sodium	

1 cup plain, low-fat or fat-free Greek yogurt

½ cup frozen orange juice concentrate, partially thawed

1. Place yogurt into a medium bowl.

2. Slowly spoon in orange concentrate, stirring slightly to give a marbling effect.

3. Place mixture into popsicle molds.

4. Freeze until firm, at least 1 hour.

GOOD MOVE

Popsicles are a great way to quench your thirst and feel like you've had a sweet treat. To insure they're not loaded with sugar make your own by freezing smoothies, fruit purées, and fruit juices.

Truffles

Dried fruit is mixed with crunchy almonds, cacao powder, and ginger, and then rolled in coconut to create a sweet, slightly bitter dessert. Take this to your next dinner party invitation.

Yield:	Serving size:	Prep time:	Cook time:
12 truffles	2 truffles	20 minutes	None

Each serving has:			
148 calories	6 g fat	26 g carbohydrates	
4 g fiber	3 g protein	3 mg sodium	

½ cup prunes, pitted

¼ cup dates, pitted

4 TB. almonds

1 TB. pure maple syrup

3 TB. raw cacao powder, unsweetened

½ TB. ginger, freshly grated

½ cup unsweetened coconut, finely grated

1. Place prunes and dates into a food processer and blend until a paste is formed, scraping down the sides as needed.

2. Blend in almonds, maple syrup, cacao powder, and ginger.

3. Roll mixture into 1-inch balls.

4. Roll balls in coconut to lightly coat the outsides.

5. Refrigerate until firm, about 1 hour.

6. Store what you don't eat in an airtight container in the refrigerator. It keeps for several weeks.

RED FLAG

While maple syrup and honey may seem like healthier sweeteners, the truth is, in the body they act just like any concentrated sugar. Use them sparingly as you would any other sweetener and you'll do fine.

Berry Crumble

Nothing beats a comforting fresh fruit crumble served warm straight from the oven. This one is topped with a healthy blend of almonds, oats, dates, and cinnamon and no added fat.

Yield:	Serving size:	Prep time:	Cook time:
6⅔ cups	⅔ cup	10 minutes	45 minutes

Each serving has:		
315 calories	10 g fat	58 g carbohydrates
10 g fiber	6 g protein	8 mg sodium

5 oz. fresh blueberries

5 oz. fresh raspberries

1 lb. fresh peaches, peeled and sliced

¼ cup fresh lemon juice

2 TB. apple juice

½ cup almonds

½ cup dry quick-cooking or old-fashioned oats

1 cup pitted, dried dates, chopped

½ tsp. cinnamon

1. Place blueberries, raspberries, and peaches in an 8-inch baking dish and cover with lemon and apple juices.

2. In a food processor, grind almonds, oats, dates, and cinnamon until they form a loose crumble.

3. Sprinkle crumble on top of fruit.

4. Bake uncovered for 45 minutes. Serve warm.

WHAT'S NEW

What's the difference between a cobbler and a crisp? Although both have a fruit base, cobblers are topped with a thick biscuit-like dough that rises in the oven, while crisps have a dry crumbly topping.

Chocolate Lover's Pie

This is a sexy pie. Smooth, rich, and decadent—and even tastier with seasonal fresh fruit like berries or peaches on the side. It's sure to be a hit at any potluck or romantic dinner.

Yield:	Serving size:	Prep time:	Cook time:
1 pie	⅛th of pie	20 minutes	30 minutes

Each serving has:		
308 calories	14 g fat	46 g carbohydrates
2 g fiber	4 g protein	109 mg sodium

1¼ cups chocolate chips	⅓ cup maple syrup
1 pkg silken tofu (12 oz.)	1 9-inch frozen pie crust, thawed
⅓ cup honey	

1. Melt chocolate chips in a double boiler.

2. Pour melted chocolate, tofu, honey, and maple syrup into a blender and blend until completely smooth.

3. Pour chocolate mixture into pie crust.

4. Bake in a 300°F oven for 20–30 minutes, until firm, but before crust browns.

5. Let cool completely, then refrigerate for at least 1 hour before serving.

GOOD MOVE

When purchasing chocolate, stick to dark chocolate with 65 percent or greater cocoa content. Dark chocolate contains far more antioxidants and health benefits than milk or white chocolate. In fact, studies show that 3.5 ounces of dark chocolate a day decreases blood pressure and lowers LDL cholesterol up to 10 percent.

Berry Parfait

Parfaits are so simple to make it's a wonder more people don't make them. Here, colorful berries are layered between creamy yogurt. Make it in a clear glass for a stunning presentation.

Yield:	Serving size:	Prep time:	Cook time:
2 cups	1 cup	5 minutes	None

Each serving has:		
236 calories	9 g fat	34 g carbohydrates
4 g fiber	8 g protein	130 mg sodium

1 cup plain, low-fat or nonfat Greek yogurt

½ cup raspberries

½ cup blueberries

½ cup granola

1. In clear glasses, layer yogurt, berries, and granola. Serve chilled.

GOOD MOVE

Blueberries are one of the few berries native to North America. There are two types: a plump, round cultivated blueberry and a small, concentrated wild blueberry. Unless you're in Maine you won't find wild berries fresh, only frozen, but they are worth the trouble—their blueberry flavor is intense and their antioxidant properties are off the charts.

Banana Colada

This tropical fruit cocktail is a great finish to any warm day, and can be a nice addition to a spicy meal as well.

Yield:	Serving size:	Prep time:	Cook time:
2 cups	1 cup	15 minutes	None

Each serving has:			
398 calories	19 g fat	61 g carbohydrates	
9 g fiber	4 g protein	14 mg sodium	

½ cup light coconut milk, canned

2 TB. lime juice

4 bananas, sliced into ¼-inch thick rounds, and then frozen

⅓ cup coconut unsweetened, finely grated

1. Place ¼ cup coconut milk into a blender with 1 tablespoon lime juice.

2. Start the blender and add frozen banana pieces, one at a time.

3. As mixture thickens, scrape down the sides of blender and add remaining coconut milk and lime juice.

4. Continue adding banana until all of it has been added and blend until all large pieces have broken down.

5. Stir in grated coconut and serve.

GOOD MOVE

Bananas are among the oldest fruits in the world. Rich in potassium and a super source of vitamin B_6, they may help reduce your risk of high blood pressure and stroke and aid your immune system.

Oatmeal Raisin Cookies

Bananas are the secret ingredient, which makes this healthful version of an oatmeal raisin cookie sweet while still being sugar-free. Enjoy!

Yield:	Serving size:	Prep time:	Cook time:
36 cookies	2 cookies	10 minutes	20 minutes

Each serving has:		
112 calories	5 g fat	17 g carbohydrates
2 g fiber	2 g protein	2 mg sodium

3 ripe bananas, peeled   ⅓ cup olive oil
2 cups rolled old-fashioned oats   1 tsp. vanilla extract
1 cup raisins

1. Preheat oven to 350°F.

2. In a large bowl, mash bananas.

3. Stir in oats, raisins, oil, and vanilla. Mix well and allow to sit for 15 minutes.

4. Drop by teaspoonfuls onto an ungreased cookie sheet.

5. Bake until golden, about 20 minutes.

RED FLAG

A serving size of cookies is two medium cookies. If you are making a large batch of homemade cookies, consider freezing most of them for a future occasion or giving them away to neighbors.

Coconut Ginger Pudding

Inspired from tapioca pudding, this dish gets its thickness from chia seeds. This "super food" is a great source of omega-3 fatty acids.

Yield:	Serving size:	Prep time:	Cook time:
1 cup	½ cup	10 minutes	15 minutes
Each serving has:			
313 calories	29 g fat	16 g carbohydrates	
3 g fiber	3 g protein	19 mg sodium	

1 cup whole milk coconut milk	1 tsp. grated ginger
1 TB. honey	1 TB. *chia* seeds

1. Place coconut milk in a medium saucepan and heat slowly over medium heat.

2. Add honey and ginger and stir until warm. Do not bring to a boil.

3. Add chia seeds and stir for another few minutes.

4. Place mixture into two tea cups or small bowls. Refrigerate until mixture becomes firm.

DEFINITION

Chia is an edible seed harvested from the plant *Salvia hispanica* and is an important food source of the Mayan people. The seed contains even more omega-3 fatty acids than flax seeds and is very rich in antioxidants. It also does not spoil nearly as easily.

Peaches and Cashew Mousse

The lightness of this mousse is a great addition to fresh peaches.

Yield:	Serving size:	Prep time:	Cook time:
4 cups	1 cup	15 minutes	None

Each serving has:			
365 calories	16 g fat	54 g carbohydrates	
5 g fiber	7 g protein	12 mg sodium	

1 cup raw cashews	½ tsp. cinnamon
½ cup water	Pinch of sea salt
2 TB. honey	1 lb. mango chunks, frozen
¼ cup orange juice concentrate	4 peaches, peeled, pitted, sliced
1 tsp. vanilla extract	

1. Place cashews in a food processor, and cover nuts with water.

2. While blending, add honey, orange juice, vanilla, cinnamon, and salt.

3. When mixed, add mango slowly to food processor until desired thickness is achieved. Add more water if necessary to make it smooth and creamy.

4. Place peach slices into bowls, top with mango cream, and serve.

GOOD MOVE

Nut butters are surprisingly simple to make and their taste is superior to commercial blends—plus you know exactly what's in them. To make, simply grind unsalted nuts in a food processor until they're a thick paste.

Getting Started with a 14-Day Menu Plan

In This Chapter

- Mastering a Mediterranean-style meal plan
- Making it work for you
- Time-saving cooking tips
- Finding menus to make your mouth water

Now that you know what to eat, what not to eat, and how much to eat to get rid of stubborn belly fat, it's time to make a plan—a menu plan. This chapter puts together all the principles you've learned to show you exactly what 14 days worth of meals should look like. Sure you could follow it exactly using the recipes included in this book, but it works best as a guide to help you get used to the meal pattern. Meal patterns are more flexible than a diet plan because they can be adjusted depending on what foods are available and what's happening in your life at the time.

Here we'll discuss the basic elements of the meal plan (foods you'll eat every day and why) and how you can adjust the diet based on season and budget. We'll also share tips, tricks, and shortcuts that save you time and money as well as keep kitchen prep work to a minimum. Because this plan is based on the Mediterranean diet, the foods you'll be eating are familiar to most people, comforting to others, and best of all, easy to find nearly anywhere in the United States. More importantly, however, is the fact that this is a way of eating that everyone in your family can enjoy—so you don't have to make another separate "meal" for the rest of the family. After you've gotten used to eating this way you'll be surprised at how delicious and easy to prepare these whole, natural, minimally processed foods can be.

Getting the Pattern Down

When most people think of the Mediterranean diet, they usually think of Italian food. It's true much of Italy (particularly southern Italy) ascribes to the Mediterranean diet, but this isn't the only cuisine that fits into this healthy eating pattern. Twenty-one countries border the Mediterranean and each one has its own unique culinary qualities. Consequently, what we call the Mediterranean diet isn't really a "diet" at all, but a traditional style of eating, shared by all these countries. This style includes eating lots of fresh vegetables and fruits, small amounts of meat, modest amounts of cheese and dairy, and seafood and shellfish at least twice a week. There are few processed foods in the diet and most of the fats are in monounsaturated form—olive oil, avocado, nuts, peanuts, and seeds. Desserts are generally fresh fruit. How does this translate into what you eat every day? Here are some of the most important points.

Nuts and Nut Butters

You'll notice in this meal plan that nuts are a staple. One to two 1-ounce servings of nuts; nut butter such as peanut, almond, or cashew butter; or seeds such as sunflower or pumpkin seeds are eaten nearly every day. The easiest way to incorporate nuts into your diet is as a snack, along with a fruit, low-fat dairy such as yogurt, or vegetables such as celery sticks. Just remember not to overdo it. One ounce is only one small handful of nuts—eat more and you'll rack up too many calories (negating some of the health benefits). In addition to snacks it's also a good idea to get used to sprinkling nuts on salads, fish, or chicken. If you don't feel like counting out nuts or are afraid your handful is bigger than it should be, buy nuts that are already proportioned in 1-ounce packages. Some even come in 100-calorie bags.

Nut milks are another great way to incorporate more nuts in your diet (soy milk is also an option) and a good alternative to whole milk, which is high in saturated fat.

What type of nut you choose depends on your own personal taste—most are interchangeable. Variety is key to a healthy diet, so try to choose as many different types of nuts as you can. The same holds true for nut and seed butters and nut milk. Here is a sampling: almonds, cashews, pistachios, peanuts, pecans, walnuts, Brazil nuts, pine nuts, sunflower seeds, pumpkin seeds, and sesame seeds.

WHAT'S NEW

Did you know macadamia nuts top the list as the nut highest in monounsaturated fat, with 17 grams per ounce and a total fat content of about 22 grams per 1 ounce? So if you do eat macadamia nuts remember to go easy on them (having only 5 or 6 at a time—about ½ ounce). The same holds true for Brazil nuts, which is next in the fat line (hold yourself to no more than 3 or 4 nuts—about ½ ounce).

Whole Grains

Whole grains are essential on the belly fat diet, not only do they increase fiber and add vital vitamins and minerals but they keep insulin levels low and specifically target belly fat. Research shows people who regularly consume whole grains (about three servings per day) have smaller waists and less belly fat than those who eat refined grains instead. As an added bonus, whole grains also reduce your risk for diabetes, metabolic syndrome, and heart disease.

In this diet plan we've kept bread intake to a minimum mostly because it eats up calories and is not as nutrient dense as whole grains. Rather you should up your intake of brown rice, quinoa, barley, and bulgur to name a few. Whole grains add taste, texture, and excitement to your meals, not to mention good nutrition. When you do eat bread, always choose whole grain instead of white and read the label to check for calories and sodium levels. Your best bet is to choose a whole-grain bread with fewer than 100 calories per slice and sodium levels no higher than 180 milligrams.

Beans and Eggs

Beans, dried peas, and lentils are staples in the Mediterranean diet and foods that most Americans don't eat nearly enough of. In this diet pattern we've included roughly 2 cups of beans, dried peas, or lentils (or more) a week in different forms. Beans can be found in salsas, salads, and hummus and as snacks mixed with herbs, spices, and cheese.

Eggs have a place in the diet, too. In fact, you can eat about three to four eggs a week on this meal plan (actually nutritionists say eating one egg a day is okay). They usually appear scrambled or hard-cooked as a snack. Super high in protein and low in calories, eggs are an ideal choice for keeping hunger at bay between meals. Although the yolk is high in cholesterol, it's low in saturated fat, high in beneficial choline, and contains plenty of fat soluble vitamins, so don't throw it out!

Fish and Shellfish

Red meat and chicken are eaten sparingly (think of them as condiments to a meal rather than the center of the plate), whereas fish and shellfish are stars. Eat them at least two times a week and more if possible. They're one of the best sources of omega-3 fatty acids in the diet. All types of fish are beneficial but the best kinds are fatty fish including salmon, trout, or tuna.

GOOD MOVE

To get the most nutritional bang for your buck try experimenting with low-cost, high-fat Mediterranean fish such as sardines, anchovies, bluefin tuna, and red mullet. Many people are surprised at how versatile and delicious they can be.

Low-Fat Dairy and Vegetarian Meals

Full-fat cheeses are okay in small amounts, but try to choose low-fat, high-quality dairy products whenever you can. Low-fat yogurt is a good example of this and plays a prominent role in the diet. If you like to drink cow's milk, choose skim or 1 percent over higher fat ones.

You should also try to squeeze in several vegetarian meals, aiming for at least two or three of these types of meals a week. Check out the recipe chapters for exciting recipe ideas.

Don't Worry About Fat

One of the biggest challenges when following this meal plan is getting over the fear of fat. Fat, especially good fat as found in peanuts, olive oil, and avocados, not only provides needed calories and protective health benefits that help release belly fat, it contributes to the enjoyment of food by giving flavor, texture, and color to meals. It's also the reason why people stick to this eating style for a lifetime.

Even with higher fat levels (Mediterranean diets can range from 30 to 40 percent of calories from fat), chances are your calorie levels still won't be too high. That's because you'll be eating more healthy, low-fat vegetables, fruits, and whole grains and you'll be keeping portion sizes small. You'll also be avoiding calorie-laden processed foods.

Calorie levels for the 14-day menu run between 1,500 and 1,900 calories, which is a good level for most active women. For men, however, you may need to bump that up a bit, particularly if you're lifting weights or playing sports. How do you know if you're not eating enough? If you're tired, fatigued, and feel hungry all the time, these are sure signs. Also, if you drop too much weight very quickly. If you do need more, here are some ways to increase calories and protein without going overboard:

- Increase nut milk to 8 ounce portions.

- Double up on vegetables. (This is the best way to increase calories.)

- Add one extra serving of nuts or nut butters to your daily meal plan.

- Increase protein by 2 ounces (totaling 6 ounces per meal).

- Add an egg to your meal plan.

If you think the calories you are eating (some people need a 1,200 to 1,400 calorie menu to start losing weight) are too high or you're not losing weight, try these tips to help slim down some meals:

- Reduce your protein intake from 4 ounce to 3 ounce portions.

- Cut your nuts and nut butters in half and replace with an extra serving of fresh fruit or vegetable.

- Drop portion sizes down from 1 cup (start with beans and grains first) to ¾ cup or ½ cup servings.

KISS—Keep It Simple Stupid

Preparation methods are easy, too, emphasizing grilled, stir-fried, baked, or broiled dishes as well as fresh salads. This will bring out the natural flavor of the food and create memorable and tasty dishes that will soon become family favorites. By avoiding fancy condiments and sauces you'll also avoid lots of salt, sugar, and excess calories.

Take a look at the recipes in Chapters 16 through 21. Many use only a handful of ingredients, some fresh herbs for flavor, and a splash of olive oil with lime juice, lemon juice, or capers for extra zing.

Reduce Your Workload

When it comes to preparing healthy food from scratch, menu planning is crucial to your success, plus it saves you tons of time and money. Using the 14-Day Menu as a guide, plan out your own menu based on what's in season and what you can afford. Write it down and use it when making your grocery list.

Buying fresh produce instead of pre-prepared means you can use that produce in many different ways. For instance, in Week 1 fennel is in the Fennel, Pear, and Romaine Lettuce Salad. It's also used in the Sautéed Shrimp and Fennel recipe for dinner, and last but not least, fresh fennel slices dipped in seasoned olive oil make a great between-meal snack. Swiss chard also shows up several times with eggs, as a bed for fish, and mixed with lentils.

Re-Tooling Leftovers

You'll also notice that recipes often appear more than once in a week. These leftovers can be a lifesaver as far as time and money management go. Rather than spend time cooking every day, think about preparing several meals in one day or, better yet, a big batch of one recipe that can be eaten throughout the week.

Take soups, for example. Soups are good food on several accounts. First, they can be made well in advance and eaten a few days later. Many times making these soups ahead of time enhances their flavor, making them taste even better later on. Second, they are extremely versatile and are a good way to use up bits and pieces of vegetables. And, finally homemade broth soups are healthy and nutritious—generally low in calories and usually packed with fiber as well as colorful vegetables and whole grains.

With a little bit of creativity and imagination, leftovers can make great lunches a day or two later. Oftentimes they can be revamped to create entirely new dishes. The Polenta with Red Sauce, for example, makes a fine Italian dinner, but mix the red sauce with ½ cup red beans, ¼ teaspoon chili powder, some shredded lettuce, and guacamole, and a few days later you've turned your Italian meal into Tex-Mex surprise.

Be Flexible

When it comes to menu planning be sure and think about seasonality and availability in your area. Mix and match beans and whole grains depending on what you can find or what you're in the mood for. Fruits, in particular, are easy to swap out. Berries are a mainstay in the diet. If fresh aren't around, look for frozen. You also might want to sub in cherries or grapes instead.

Take the same approach with vegetables. Stay attuned to the season focusing on root vegetables, cabbage, broccoli, and cauliflower in the cold winter months; asparagus and leafy greens in the Spring; zucchini, peppers, and tomatoes in the Summer; and squash, onions, kale, beets, and potatoes in the Fall.

Greens in particular can be easily substituted. Lettuces come in all sizes and colors, although dark leafy green lettuces are best. If you want iceberg instead of romaine, green leaf lettuce, or Boston Bibb go ahead, just make sure to get your veggie quota elsewhere.

Cooking greens are just as adaptable. Don't have Swiss chard? Try using spinach instead, or else arugula or beet greens. You may even want to combine some greens together. Although they each bring a different flavor profile, after you get the hang of it, it will be easy to create satisfying and interesting meals.

14-Day Menu Plan

Week 1

DAY 1
1,733 calories, 68 g fat, 207 g carbohydrates, 36 g fiber, 81 g protein, 1,631 mg sodium

Breakfast	***Wilted Chard and Eggs***
	1 cup sliced strawberries
	6 oz. nut milk
Snack	***Hummus with Vegetables***
Lunch	4 oz. broiled chicken breast topped with ***Festive Roasted Peppers***
	1 cup cooked barley mixed with 2 TB. chopped almonds, 1 tsp. olive oil, and 1 TB. chopped parsley
Snack	***Berry Parfait***
Dinner	***Chickpea and Rice Stew***
	2 cups romaine lettuce, ½ tomato and ½ cucumber, sliced and dressed with 1 tsp. olive oil and 1 tsp. balsamic vinegar

DAY 2
1,546 calories, 52 g fat, 240 g carbohydrates, 38 g fiber, 57 g protein, 1,478 mg sodium

Breakfast	***Cottage Cheese and Melon*** sprinkled with 1 TB. sunflower seeds and ¼ tsp. cinnamon
Snack	1 apple, sliced
	7 walnut halves
Lunch	***Fish Tacos***
	1½ cups steamed green beans
	6 oz. nut milk
Snack	8 celery sticks and 8 carrot sticks
	1½ TB. almond butter
Dinner	***Polenta with Red Sauce***
	2 cups Swiss chard, sautéed with 1 tsp. olive oil and 1 small chopped onion
	1 pear

DAY 3
1,671 calories, 65 g fat, 218 g carbohydrates, 49 g fiber, 75 g protein, 1,285 mg sodium

Breakfast	¾ cup cooked old-fashioned oatmeal mixed with 1 cup blueberries, 4 oz. almond or any nut milk, and 1 tsp. honey
Snack	1 cup **Butternut Squash Soup** sprinkled with ¼ cup chopped pistachios
Lunch	**Black Bean Salad** in a whole-wheat tortilla topped with 2 slices avocado
Snack	1 cup raspberries
	1 low-fat mozzarella stick
Dinner	4 oz. roasted cod topped with 1 tsp. pesto
	1 large baked sweet potato
	Spicy Sautéed Broccoli

DAY 4
1,796 calories, 74 g fat, 199 g carbohydrates, 41 g fiber, 93 g protein, 1,749 mg sodium

Breakfast	¾ cup plain, low-fat yogurt topped with 1 cup strawberries and ¼ cup low-fat granola
Snack	1 hard-cooked egg
	½ oz. whole almonds (about 12)
Lunch	**Fennel, Pear, and Romaine Salad with Vinaigrette** with 6 large broiled shrimp, ½ cup cooked chickpeas, and ½ oz. feta cheese
Snack	**Hummus with Vegetables**
Dinner	**Tandoori Chicken**
	¾ cup cooked brown rice
	Lentils with Swiss Chard
	1 small apple

DAY 5
1,661 calories, 50 g fat, 253 g carbohydrates, 38 g fiber, 66 g protein, 1,663 mg sodium

Breakfast	***Oatmeal Parfait***
	4 oz. nut milk
Snack	5 whole-grain sesame seed crackers with 1 TB. peanut butter
	1 pear
Lunch	***Polenta with Red Sauce***
	½ cup black beans sprinkled with ¼ tsp. chili powder and ¾ cup blueberries
Snack	½ cup plain, low-fat yogurt topped with 6 whole, chopped almonds and ½ tsp. honey
Dinner	3 oz. Broiled Salmon topped with ***Festive Roasted Peppers***
	½ cup cooked barley
	Lemony Kale

DAY 6
1,680 calories, 54 g fat, 197 g carbohydrates, 39 g fiber, 116 g protein, 1,681 mg sodium

Breakfast	2 eggs, scrambled, ***Black Bean Salad,*** and 1 slice avocado, wrapped in a whole-wheat tortilla
Snack	1 baked sweet potato drizzled with ½ tsp. olive oil, 7 walnut halves (chopped), and a sprinkle of cinnamon and cayenne
Lunch	3 oz. tuna, mixed with ½ cup plain, nonfat Greek yogurt, ½ TB. sunflower seeds, ½ apple (chopped), ½ celery stick (chopped), and ½ carrot (chopped), served on 2 cups torn romaine lettuce
Snack	1 cup mixed berries
	1 low-fat mozzarella stick
Dinner	***Sautéed Shrimp and Fennel***
	1 cup broccoli with squeeze of lemon
	¾ cup brown rice

DAY 7
1,577 calories, 69 g fat, 175 g carbohydrates, 44 g fiber, 86 g protein, 1,520 mg sodium

Breakfast	1 cup high-fiber, low-sugar cereal (try Kashi or Cascadian Farm brands)
	4 oz. nut milk
Snack	***Hummus with Vegetables***
	5 whole-grain sesame crackers (try Ak-Mak)
Lunch	***Butternut Squash Soup,*** topped with 1 TB. pistachios, chopped
	Fennel, Pear, and Romaine Salad with Vinaigrette, topped with ½ oz. feta cheese
Snack	6 carrot sticks and 6 celery sticks
	1 TB. almond butter mixed with 2 TB. plain, nonfat Greek yogurt
Dinner	4 oz. broiled sirloin steak (sliced) served over a salad of 3 cups romaine lettuce, 1 small tomato (sliced), ½ cucumber (sliced), ½ cup cooked corn, and ½ small red onion (sliced), dressed with 1 tsp. olive oil, 1 tsp. balsamic vinegar, salt, and pepper

Week 2

DAY 8
1,575 calories, 72 g fat, 173 g carbohydrates, 27 g fiber, 75 g protein, 1,150 mg sodium

Breakfast	***Tropical Smoothie***
	1 hard-cooked egg
Snack	2 TB. nut butter (cashew, peanut, or almond)
	6 whole-grain crackers
Lunch	***Chicken Caesar Salad***
	1 apple
Snack	6 oz. nut milk
	10 grapes or cherries
Dinner	***Seared Scallops***
	1 cup roasted carrots
	Tomato salad, made up of 1 tomato, sliced and topped with 3 torn basil leaves, 1 tsp. olive oil, salt, and pepper *(option: double the recipe and save half for Day 11)*

DAY 9
1,741 calories, 71 g fat, 208 g carbohydrates, 40 g fiber, 95 g protein, 1,061 mg sodium

Breakfast	1 cup high-fiber, low-sugar whole-grain cereal (try Kashi or Cascadian Farms brands)
	6 oz. nut milk
	1 small peach, sliced
Snack	*Tropical Smoothie*
	7 walnut halves
Lunch	*Tomato Basil Soup*
	3 oz. broiled Tilapia with 2 lemon slices
Snack	19 pecan halves
	½ mango, sliced
Dinner	3 oz. broiled pork tenderloin
	2 cups steamed cauliflower topped with 2 tsp. grated Parmesan cheese, 1 tsp. chopped parsley, 1 tsp. olive oil, and pepper
	Summer Quinoa Salad

DAY 10
1,569 calories, 50 g fat, 241 g carbohydrates, 54 g fiber, 63 g protein, 1,605 mg sodium

Breakfast	1 cup cooked old-fashioned oatmeal mixed with 2 TB. peanut butter, 1 cup sliced strawberries or grapes, 6 oz. nut milk, 1 tsp. honey
Snack	*Trail Mix*
	1 apple
Lunch	*Pita Salad Sandwich*
	1 cup blackberries
Snack	½ red pepper sliced
	1 low-fat mozzarella stick
Dinner	*Saffron Bulgur* mixed with 1 cup cooked red beans

DAY 11
1,683 calories, 67 g fat, 180 g carbohydrates, 39 g fiber, 99 g protein, 1,535 mg sodium

Breakfast	2 eggs scrambled with ½ small tomato (chopped), and ½ onion (chopped), sautéed in 1 tsp. olive oil, served in ½ whole-wheat pita
Snack	*Tomato Basil Soup* topped with ¾ cup cooked white beans
Lunch	3 oz. broiled salmon topped with ½ mango (diced), mixed with 1 TB. chopped cilantro, 2 tsp. olive oil, ½ lime squeezed, served on 4 cups raw spinach leaves
Snack	*Summer Quinoa Salad*
	½ oz. feta
Dinner	*Lemon Caper Chicken*
	2 cups steamed green beans
	Tomato salad, made of 1 tomato, sliced and topped with 3 torn basil leaves, 1 tsp. olive oil, salt, and pepper

DAY 12
1,747 calories, 79 g fat, 179 g carbohydrates, 32 g fiber, 100 g protein, 1,680 mg sodium

Breakfast	1 cup plain, nonfat or low-fat Greek yogurt, mixed with ½ banana, mashed, ¼ cup unsalted peanuts, 1 TB. peanut butter, dash of cinnamon
Snack	2 cups cubed papaya, topped with 2 mint leaves, shredded
Lunch	*Chopped Niçoise Salad*
	10 pecan halves
Snack	1 slice *Chocolate Lover's Pie*
	1 cup raspberries
Dinner	*Steamed Mussels with Lemongrass*
	1 whole-wheat roll

DAY 13
1,689 calories, 79 g fat, 206 g carbohydrates, 34 g fiber, 59 g protein, 1,505 mg sodium

Breakfast	¼ cup cashew or other nut butter, mixed with ½ mashed banana on 6 whole-wheat crackers
	6 oz. nut milk
Snack	*Trail Mix*
	10 grapes
Lunch	*Pita Salad Sandwich* or *Saffron Bulgur*
	1 cup raspberries
Snack	1 hard-cooked egg, topped with ½ oz. Parmesan cheese
Dinner	Tofu stir fry, made up of 4 oz. tofu, 1 cup zucchini (shredded), 1 cup carrot (shredded), and 3 cups raw spinach, sautéed with 1 tsp. sesame seed oil and 1 tsp. low-sodium soy sauce
	1 cup brown rice

DAY 14
1,673 calories, 67 g fat, 205 g carbohydrates, 37 g fiber, 77 g protein, 1,220 mg sodium

Breakfast	*Oatmeal Parfait*
Snack	1 apple
	1 TB. almond or nut butter
Lunch	*Stuffed Grape Leaves*
	1 cup cooked white beans
	10 grapes or cherries
Snack	6 oz. nut milk
	19 pecan halves
Dinner	*Zesty Steak*
	Summer Quinoa Salad
	1 cup steamed green beans

The Least You Need to Know

- The Mediterranean diet is a flexibile diet that emphasizes eating fresh vegetables and fruits, small amounts of meat, modest amounts of cheese and dairy, and seafood and shellfish at least twice a week.

- You can adapt any cuisine or eating lifestyle to the Mediterranean eating plan and lifestyle.

- The best way to stick to your meal plan is to plan out menus ahead of time.

- To maximize your meal plans and save time and money, keep it simple, use leftovers, and prepare foods ahead of time.

- It takes only a few small changes to decrease calories in your diet.

Glossary

adrenaline   A fast-acting peptide hormone released by the adrenal glands and nervous system in an acute stress response. It causes an abrupt, sometimes extreme elevation of heart rate and blood pressure, cold hands and feet, and sweating.

alpha waves   A pattern of electrical activity in the brain that's associated with relaxation and is suppressed during times of stress.

anchovies   Small fish that are cured in such a way to create a strong, pungent taste—a savory garnish for salads and grains.

arugula   A spicy, peppery salad green that is part of the mustard family, and high in fat-soluble vitamins A and K.

autonomic nervous system (ANS)   The part of the nervous system that controls involuntary bodily functions, and specifically internal organs such as smooth muscles in the heart, blood vessels, and digestive organs; glands such as the salivary, gastric, and sweat glands; and the adrenals. It's divided into two subsystems: the sympathetic nervous system, which kicks in, in response to stress, and the parasympathetic nervous system, which is calming and relaxing.

basal metabolic rate (BMR)   The number of kilocalories per day your body requires to maintain all vital functions when you're at rest.

belly fat   A unique type of adipose tissue (fat) that accumulates inside the abdomen. You don't have to be overweight to have belly fat. This type of fat is a major risk factor for diabetes, heart disease, and other chronic illnesses.

blood pressure   The force with which your heart pumps blood to the body—stress-related elevations in blood pressure can increase your risk of developing heart disease and stroke.

body mass index (BMI)   A calculation of height and weight used to determine if a person is overweight. A drawback of this method is that it does not take body composition (for example, muscle mass) into consideration.

boiling   Method of cooking where food is placed in water heated to a temperature of 212°F. Bubbles break the surface. Best used with vegetables.

bulgur   Whole wheat that is first steamed or parboiled, dried, and then crushed or ground. It is a staple in Middle Eastern cuisine and is an inexpensive source of low-fat protein.

cacao   The raw, unprocessed beans of the cocoa plant that have a rich, intense flavor. Rich in antioxidants.

caffeine   A stimulant found in coffee, tea, and cola products. It revs up metabolism, boosting energy and alertness. Too much can cause heart palpitations, shakiness, jitters, and sleeplessness.

capers   The young flower bud of a caper plant that is then pickled and cured in salt or a salt-vinegar solution. During the curing process, the caper releases mustard oil, which gives it that distinct, intense flavor, similar to green olives.

cardiovascular reactivity   The elevation in heart rate and blood pressure that occurs in response to an event, situation, or thought that's perceived to be threatening.

chia   The edible seed from the salvia plant that is very rich in omega-3 fatty acids.

cholesterol   A type of lipid produced by the liver and used by the body for producing steroid hormones and maintaining cell membranes. Too much cholesterol contributes to heart disease. Cholesterol is found only in animal and animal products, including fish.

complex carbohydrates   Large chains of simple sugars produced by plants, including fiber and starch.

coping   The things a person thinks and does to try to feel better when life becomes stressful or overwhelming.

cortisol   Secreted by the adrenal gland during times of stress, cortisol is a hormone that shifts metabolism toward energy conservation and fat storage. It stimulates appetite, induces cravings for fatty, sugary foods, and promotes belly fat.

cruciferous vegetables   Vegetables which have a cross-shaped flower, found in the cabbage and mustard family, include broccoli, cauliflower, kale, and arugula to name a few. They've been shown to provide protection against oxidative damage and cancer.

curry powder   A blend of spices, many of which have strong antioxidant ability, used in many Indian and Asian dishes.

diet   The food and beverages a person eats and drinks on a daily basis.

dietary fiber   Structural components of plant-based food that remain after exposure to digestive enzymes and acids.

disaccharide   A sugar that is composed of two monosaccharide molecules, such as sucrose, which is made of one molecule of glucose and one molecule of fructose.

drink (alcoholic)   A single "drink" of an alcoholic beverage is defined as 12 ounces of beer, 5 ounces of wine, or 1.5 ounces of distilled spirits.

elliptical trainer   An exercise machine found in most gyms that provides a strenuous workout with minimal impact on joints.

emotional regulation   A type of coping that a person does to soothe anxiety or other negative emotions in response to perceived stress.

essential fatty acids   Long-chain fat molecules that the human body can't synthesize, and thus requires from food. Examples include linoleic and alpha-linolenic acids.

exercise   Strenuous physical activity that enhances physical fitness and reduces the risk of disease. Distinct from general physical activity in that it is specifically planned, structured, and repetitive.

fad diets   Popular eating plans that promise quick weight loss by severely limiting food intake and/or the consumption of certain foods while overemphasizing others. Fad diets don't work long term.

fennel bulbs   Celery-like food with a mild licorice flavor commonly used in Mediterranean cuisine; high in beneficial phytonutrients.

fiber   The non-starchy complex carbohydrates that make up the structural components of plants. Some types of fiber are digestible by humans, and some, such as cellulose, are not. They promote good health by slowing absorption of sugars in the diet, absorbing fat and cholesterol in the intestines, and protecting against constipation.

fructose   A monosaccharide that is found in fruits, some vegetables, and honey. It is the sweetest naturally occurring sugar.

genes   Stretches of DNA that code for all manner of individual characteristics such as hair color, height, etc.

glucose   The major monosaccharide found in blood, serving as an energy source for all cells in the body; found in fruits, sweet corn, corn syrup, honey, and certain root vegetables such as beets.

glycogen   A large molecule characterized by its branched structure, made by the liver and skeletal muscle out of glucose molecules for energy storage.

grains   Small fruit that's found on grassy crops such as wheat, oats, rice, and barley. Each kernel of whole grain has a tough outer coating called the bran, which is rich in fiber and essential fatty acids. The endosperm is located inside the whole grain, and is rich in starch and protein. The germ makes up the bottom of the whole grain and is high in fat.

grape leaves   A type of leaf traditionally used in Greek, Turkish, Bulgarian, and Arab cuisines. They are most often picked fresh, stuffed with a mixture of rice, vegetables, and spices, and cooked by boiling or steaming. In the United States, fresh grape leaves are hard to find. Most often you'll see them brined in a can or jar.

high fructose corn syrup (HFCS)   A highly processed sweetener extracted from corn and composed of a combination of fructose and glucose, HFCS has been implicated in elevating one's risk of fatty deposits in the liver and insulin resistance.

high-density lipoprotein (HDL)   A large particle composed of proteins and fats (lipids) that function to transport cholesterol from the body's cells and tissues back to the liver for excretion in the bile. Known as the "good cholesterol." HDL should be greater than 60 mg/dL to be protective against cardiovascular disease.

human growth hormone (HGH)   Highest in children, HGH increases muscle development and decreases fat. As we age, HGH levels decrease but regular physical activity can turn that around and actually raise HGH levels. Found in most processed foods.

hydrogenated or partially hydrogenated fats   Man-made fats which are created by bombarding vegetable oil with hydrogen, turning the liquid fat into a solid, thus giving it a longer shelf life for use in processed foods.

impaired glucose tolerance (IGT)   A pre-diabetic condition in which blood sugar levels are elevated because the body's insulin receptors have become less responsive to insulin. This happens most often in people who are overweight, obese, or have large amounts of belly fat.

inactivity physiology   The study of the effects of sedentariness on metabolism and risk factors for chronic disease.

insoluble fiber   Fiber that doesn't dissolve in water and therefore isn't digested and absorbed in the human body. Found in beans, whole grains, cabbage, and broccoli, insoluble fiber has been found to be protective against colon cancer.

instant oats   Similar to quick-cooking oats except these oats are cut in pieces; flavoring ingredients are usually added.

insulin   A steroid hormone secreted by the pancreas in response to high blood sugar levels. Insulin allows muscle and fat cells to use glucose (blood sugar) for energy and for storing as fat.

insulin resistance   The underlying dysfunction in Type 2 diabetes, this is a condition in which cells have a lower than normal response to insulin, meaning it takes more insulin for cells to utilize glucose. Insulin resistance tends to occur in people who are overweight, especially with belly fat.

legumes   Legumes are a class of vegetables that include beans, peas, lentils, and peanuts. They are high in protein and a good source of vitamins and minerals.

lemongrass   Lemongrass is a long, thin stalk with a light lemony flavor, often paired with garlic, lime, cilantro, or chilies. It is common in Thai, Indian, and Vietnamese dishes.

limbic system   The part of the brain that is involved with emotions and motivations at a primitive, frequently survival-oriented level.

lipoproteins   Particles made by the liver that contain protein, triglycerides, cholesterol, and other molecules for transport through the bloodstream to the cells.

low-density lipoprotein (LDL)   A large particle composed of proteins and fats (lipids) that carries cholesterol from the liver to the tissues of the body. Elevated levels are a risk factor for heart disease; aim to keep LDL levels between 70 and 100 mg/dL.

Mediterranean diet   Traditional diet eaten by the people who live around the Mediterranean Sea; it is high in fruits, vegetables, beans, omega-3 fatty acids, and grains, and contains moderate amounts of meat, cheese, dairy, and wine.

metabolism   The process of using energy to carry out all the basic functions of life.

monounsaturated fats (MUFAs)   A type of naturally occurring fat, containing double bonds, that is found in high levels in avocado, nuts, olives, and seeds. MUFAs are used by the body to build and maintain healthy, fluid cell membranes.

nighttime-eating syndrome   A type of unhealthy eating that's characterized by eating more than 25 percent of your calories after a normal dinner time and/or getting out of bed to eat during the night at least three times per week.

normal weight obesity   This is a condition where poor diet and a sedentary lifestyle lead to excess body fat around the belly even in people who appear to be thin and maintain a healthy weight.

obesity   Having a BMI higher than 30. Usually this means weighing 20 percent or more above normal body weight.

overweight   Having a BMI between 25 and 29, usually this means weighing 10 percent above normal body weight.

palatability   The quality of food that makes it pleasant to eat and highly desirable. Highly palatable foods tend to be sweet and/or fatty, but this can vary from person to person. Palatable food tends to trigger overeating.

Paleolithic or Paleo diet   The type of diet man subsisted on before agriculture, mainly through hunting and gathering food, wild plants, and animals. Rich in meat, nuts, and seeds.

parasympathetic nervous system   The division of the autonomic nervous system that originates in the cervical and sacral spine, sending fibers throughout the body that induces relaxation of skeletal muscle, and slowing of heart and respiratory rates, as well as lowering blood pressure.

pesto   A traditional Mediterranean sauce made of oil, garlic, and whole-leaf herbs—usually basil.

physical activity   Any bodily movement, generally done in the course of one's everyday life at home or work, that involves the skeletal muscles and uses more energy than sitting or lying still.

phytonutrients   A broad array of beneficial nutrients found only in plants that have been found to help prevent oxidative damage to cells.

Pilates   A system of core-strengthening exercises developed by Joseph Pilates that helps prevent back pain, promote good posture, and tone and tighten the abdominal muscles.

pita bread   A type of unleavened bread used in many traditional dishes from Turkey and Greece. It is often used to scoop dips such as hummus, or to wrap falafel, and can be found in both white and whole-wheat forms in most grocery stores.

poaching   A gentle cooking method where food is cooked in liquid heated to 160°F to 180°F, which means the water barely shows signs of bubbles.

polenta   A paste made from ground cornmeal boiled in water. Polenta can be soft and creamy or firm and dry and is a staple of northern Italian cuisine.

polyunsaturated fats (PUFAs)   A type of fat found in fish and plants, many of which are beneficial for health. Omega-3 and omega-6 fatty acids are PUFAs.

problem management   A type of coping in the face of stress that's aimed at finding solutions to the problems and challenges that cause stress.

processed foods   Foods that have been treated to change their physical, chemical, microbiological, or sensory properties, usually to enhance palatability or to lengthen shelf life.

protein   Proteins are large molecules made up of amino acids that provide structure to tissues such as skin and bones. Other proteins function as enzymes, regulating all metabolic processes.

pulses   Grain legumes, grown primarily for their seeds, including beans, lentils, peas, and peanuts.

quick-cooking oats   Rolled oats that are flattened, making them thinner and faster to cook.

quinoa   A whole grain native to South America and a staple of traditional diets. Quinoa is one of the few plant foods to contain all nine essential amino acids (proteins) needed by the body. It has a nutty taste and is excellent used in place of rice.

refined grains   Grains that have had the fibrous bran and nutritious germ stripped from them, leaving only the starchy endosperm behind. Refined carbohydrates include white flour, white sugar, and white rice.

refined sugars   Simple carbohydrates extracted from natural sources such as sugar cane and beets. White table sugar, cane sugar, and high fructose corn syrup are refined sugars.

resistin   A hormone produced by abdominal fat that causes insulin resistance and leads to weight gain around the belly.

rolled oats or old fashioned oats   Whole oat kernels that are steamed and then flattened by rollers and dried into flakes. Take longer to cook than instant oat varieties.

root vegetables   Plant roots that are edible and flavorful and contain high levels of beneficial phytonutrients.

salt   A natural flavoring ingredient composed of 40 percent sodium and 60 percent chloride. Sodium enhances palatability, and tends to be present in excessive amounts in processed food. Aim to keep sodium levels below 2,300 milligrams per day.

satiation   The sensation of having eaten enough to satisfy hunger, signaling that it's time to stop eating.

satiety   The feeling of fullness and satisfaction that one feels between meals.

saturated fats   Type of fat that's solid at room temperature, contains single bonds, and is found only in animal foods such as meat, dairy, fish, and eggs. Some types of saturated fat contribute to belly fat, heart disease, and other illnesses.

simmering   Cooking food in liquid heated to a temperature of 185°F to 205°F; bubbles form on the bottom and rise to the top, but it is not yet boiling.

simple sugars   Single or double-chain sugars readily absorbed by the body. In food the main ones are sucrose (table sugar), fructose (fruit sugar), maltose, and lactose.

soluble fiber   Dissolves in water and is found in fruits, vegetables, beans, and oats. Soluble fiber is also found in pectin and gum. It slows digestion and helps you to better absorb nutrients from food.

sorbitol   A sugar alcohol that occurs naturally in some fruits, frequently used to sweeten "sugar-free" foods.

steel-cut oats   Whole oat kernels (known as oat groats) that have been cut in small pieces by a steel blade.

stress   The state arising when the individual perceives that the demands placed on them exceed (or threaten to exceed) their capacity to cope, and therefore threaten their well-being.

sucrose   Ordinary table sugar—found in sugar cane, sugar beets, molasses, maple syrup, fruit, vegetables, and honey—comprised of one molecule of glucose bonded to one molecule of fructose.

sympathetic nervous system   The division of the autonomic nervous system with cells in the thoracic and lumbar segments of the spinal cord that secrete molecules to induce stress-related activity such as increased heart rate and blood pressure, and shunting of blood away from the skin and digestive organs, to the head and skeletal muscles.

tahini   Sesame seed paste, commonly added to chickpeas in hummus.

tamari   A type of soy sauce that is wheat free, with a richer flavor than regular soy sauce.

trans fats   A type of fat created by partially hydrogenating or hydrogenating fats. In the body, trans fats are more dangerous than saturated fats and promote belly fat, heart disease, and other chronic illnesses. Found in many processed foods.

triglyceride   A fat molecule that consists of three fatty acids bonded to a water-soluble glycerol molecule for transport and storage in the body. Aim to keep triglyceride levels below 150 mg/dL.

Type 1 diabetes   A condition where the pancreas is unable to produce insulin at all, resulting in cells that cannot take up glucose, leading to high blood sugar levels, fatigue, malnutrition, and eventually death.

Type 2 diabetes   A condition that occurs gradually, where cells become less and less responsive to insulin resulting in higher and higher blood sugar levels and the inability of the body to handle carbohydrates. Type 2 diabetes can usually be controlled by diet and exercise, whereas Type 1 diabetes needs insulin injections.

vagus nerve   A cranial nerve, central to the parasympathetic nervous system, which innervates structures from the head down to the lower abdomen. Stimulation of the vagus nerve results in body-wide relaxation and optimal digestive function as well as increased brain levels of the neurotransmitters serotonin and dopamine.

yogurt   A type of fermented milk that originated in Turkey more than a thousand years ago. True yogurt contains "probiotics," or good bacteria, that can help promote a healthy digestive track and even boost your immune system. Many individuals that are lactose-intolerant find that they can tolerate yogurt.

Resources

In this appendix, you'll find some great books and websites that provide resources and information to support your lean belly plan and help you along the way. These are all sources that we use in our work with students and clients—and for ourselves—so we know they're reliable and useful.

Tools for the Program

Body Mass Index (BMI) Calculator (www.cdc.gov/healthyweight/assessing/bmi)—A resource provided by the Centers for Disease Control and Prevention.

Waist-Hip Ratio Calculator (www.healthfinder.gov/docs/doc11858.htm)—Calculator and other resources from the U.S. Department of Health & Human Services.

Guided Imagery

Rossman, Martin. *Guided Imagery for Self-Healing.* Novato, CA: HJ Kramer/New World Library, 2000. Dr. Rossman is a leading guided imagery teacher. This book provides a helpful overview of imagery and a wide selection of specific scripts that can be used for stress management and dealing with particular conditions.

Academy for Guided Imagery (acadgi.com/index.html)—AGI offers a comprehensive curriculum for teaching Interactive Guided Imagery skills to health professionals. The site contains basic information about guided imagery and a directory of imagery practitioners.

Belleruth Naparstek's Health Journeys (www.healthjourneys.com)—Website chock-full of news and resources from one of the leading experts in guided imagery.

Weight Loss and Management Resources

Livestrong (www.livestrong.com)—Founded by Lance Armstrong, Livestrong provides tools to track your diet, exercise, and lifestyle changes (such as quitting smoking). Lots of good nutrition, diet, and health information.

SparkPeople (www.sparkpeople.com)—A website designed to help people lose weight and promote healthy lifestyles. Includes many tools, reports, diet logs, and a strong community to keep people motivated.

The National Weight Control Registry (www.nwcr.ws)—The NWCR is a large research project begun in 1994 to study the characteristics and behaviors of more than 5,000 people who have achieved long-term successful weight-loss maintenance. This project has yielded lots of useful information for people who want to lose weight and keep it off.

WIN: Weight-Control Information Network (win.niddk.nih.gov/index.htm)—An informational site provided by the National Institutes of Health.

Meditation

Nhat Hanh, Thich. *The Miracle of Mindfulness: An Introduction to the Practice of Meditation.* Boston, MA: Beacon Press, 1976. Nhat Hanh is a Vietnamese Buddhist monk who has been teaching mindfulness meditation to people from all walks of life for more than 40 years. This little book is an excellent introduction to the philosophy and practice of mindfulness.

Shambhala (www.shambhala.org)—A global community of meditation centers and groups that are based in Tibetan Buddhism. Mindfulness meditation instruction is offered free of charge at their centers to anyone, regardless of religious or spiritual background.

Stress Management and Mind-Body Medicine

Borysenko, Joan. *Minding the Body, Mending the Mind.* Reading, MA: Addison-Wesley Publishing, 1987. This book is a classic—written by a pioneer in the field of mind-body medicine, it's engaging, informative, and full of practical, use-today ideas.

Gordon, James. *Unstuck: Your Guide to the Seven-Stage Journey Out of Depression.* New York, NY: The Penguin Press, 2008. Dr. Gordon, the founder and director of the Center for Mind-Body Medicine, presents an integrative, compassionate, and powerfully effective approach for healing depression.

Sapolsky, Robert. *Why Zebras Don't Get Ulcers.* New York, NY: Henry Holt Publishers, 2004. This book is an engaging, fun read about the many ways stress affects health, written by one of the world's leading stress researchers.

Wheeler, Claire. *10 Simple Solutions to Stress.* Oakland, CA: New Harbinger Publishers, 2007. Based in mind-body medicine, this book provides ten unique skills for managing the effects of stress that anyone can learn.

Benson-Henry Institute for Mind Body Medicine (www.massgeneral.org/bhi)— Founded by Herbert Benson, MD, the institute offers MBM programs for people with medical conditions and stress management.

The Center for Mind-Body Medicine (www.cmbm.org)—This organization has trained thousands of health professionals in the use of MBM in a wide variety of settings. Their website is rich with information and listings of MBM practitioners.

Yogafinder (www.yogafinder.com)—This is the world's largest online directory for finding yoga classes, instructors, retreats, and products.

Mindful Eating

Wansink, Brian. *Mindless Eating: Why We Eat More Than We Think.* New York, NY: Bantam Dell, 2006. Wansink is the nation's foremost expert on how our eating habits are affected by the people, places, and things in everyday life—and how to take more control over what, when, and how you eat.

The Center for Mindful Eating (www.tcme.org)—Their website provides extensive information about the research on mindful eating and how to incorporate it into everyday life.

Nutrition and Diet

Bennion, Marion and Barbara Scheule. *Introductory Foods*, Thirteenth Edition. Upper Saddle River, NJ: Prentice Hall, 2009. This book explains basic food principles from a food science perspective, giving you the why as well as the how to make sauces, muffins, breads, and more. Great for beginners.

Nestle, Marion. *What to Eat*. New York, NY: North Point Press, 2006. This detailed, well-researched, and comprehensive book is an invaluable guide to finding what's good and what to avoid at the supermarket.

Pollan, Michael. *Food Rules: An Eater's Manual*. New York, NY: Penguin Books, 2009. Based on Pollan's three rules of nutrition (eat food, mostly plants, not too much), this little book is rich in simple, straightforward advice on eating healthfully.

Tessmer, Kimberly A. and Stephanie Green. *The Complete Idiot's Guide to the Mediterranean Diet*. Indianapolis, IN: Alpha Books, 2010. This book explains clearly and thoroughly what the Mediterranean diet is (it's actually a lifestyle) and how to make it your own with meal plans and recipes.

Whitney, Eleanor Noss and Sharon Rady Rolfes. *Understanding Nutrition*, Twelfth Edition. Belmont, CA: Wadsworth Thomson Learning, 2011. This basic nutrition book tells you everything you need to know about fats, carbohydrates, protein, vitamins, and minerals throughout the lifecycle.

Labensky, Sarah R., Priscilla R. Martel, and Alan M. Hause. *On Cooking: A Textbook of Culinary Fundamentals*, Fifth Edition. Upper Saddle River: Prentice Hall, 2010. This comprehensive guide explores cooking ingredients, method, history, equipment, tools, and science. There's even a chapter on healthy cooking.

Popkin, Barry M. *The World Is Fat*. New York, NY: Avery, 2009. Popkin is a professor at University of North Carolina who specializes in global nutrition. This book takes you around the world and back again to discuss the fads, trends, policies, and products that are fattening the human race.

Welland, Diane A. *The Complete Idiot's Guide to Eating Clean*. Indianapolis, IN: Alpha Books, 2009. Learn how to ditch processed foods and create amazing dishes using whole, all-natural foods. This book shows readers how easy it is to change their eating habits one step at a time, without breaking their budgets or sacrificing taste.

Wolf, Robb. *The Paleo Solution: The Original Human Diet*. Auberry, CA: Victory Belt Publishing, 2010. This comprehensive guide book details the what, why, and how of the Paleo diet, written by an athlete turned biochemist.

Cooking Light magazine (www.cookinglight.com)—Making healthy taste great.

Eating Well magazine (www.eatingwell.com)—Where good taste meets good health.

Environmental Nutrition (www.environmentalnutrition.com)—A nutrition newsletter dedicated to informing health professionals and foodies about the newest nutrition research.

Nutrition Action HealthLetter (www.cspinet.org)—Published by the Center for Science in the Public Interest, a watchdog organization devoted to improving public health.

Tufts University Health & Nutrition Letter (www.tuftshealthletter.com)—Covers current health and nutrition diet trends and research.

University of California Berkley Wellness Letter (www.wellnessletter.com)—The newsletter of nutrition, fitness, and self-care.

Weill Cornell Medical College Health Newsletters Women's Health Advisor (www. cornellwomenshealth.com/health_information/health_newsletters.html)—A food and fitness advisor.

Online Health and Nutrition Information

American Heart Association (www.americanheart.org)—National group devoted to reducing cardiovascular disease and stroke by promoting healthy lifestyles, nutrition, and diet.

MayoClinic (www.mayoclinic.com)—Health information provided by doctors, scientists, dietitians, and health practitioners from the renowned Mayo Clinic in Rochester, Minnesota.

Medicinenet.com (www.medicinenet.com)—Bringing doctor's knowledge to you, this website is devoted to providing detailed health care, medical, and nutrition information to the general public.

MyPlate (www.choosemyplate.gov)—Guidance on how to put the USDA dietary guidelines into practice.

USDA Dietary Guidelines (www.dietaryguidelines.gov)—The federal government's evidence-based nutritional guidance to promote health, reduce the risk of chronic diseases, and reduce the prevalence of people who are overweight or obese through improved nutrition and physical activity.

Oldways (www.oldwayspt.org)—A non-profit group dedicated to preserving the "oldways" of drinking, eating, serving, and enjoying food; a big promoter of the Mediterranean diet.

WebMD (www.webmd.com)—One of the best sources of health information online, written by doctors, dietitians, journalists, and health professionals, the articles are reviewed by a medical board.

Online Food and Fitness Journals

DailyBurn (www.dailyburn.com)—Provides fitness plans, nutrition tracking, and social motivation. This site even has a scanner app, so all you need to do is scan a food's bar code with your phone to track it in your log.

FitDay (www.fitday.com)—Provides a free diet and weight-loss journal to track the foods you have eaten, daily exercise, current weight, and weight-loss goals.

MyFoodDiary.com (www.myfooddiary.com)—A data management website designed for people who want to lose weight and get healthier. It's a great tool for self-monitoring, with food and exercise logs, progress reports, and a member forum for support.

Online Calorie Calculators and Weight-Loss Programs

Free Dieting (www.freedieting.com)—Tells you how many calories you need to eat to maintain or lose weight.

MayoClinic (www.mayoclinic.com)—Based on age, height, weight, and activity level, the calculator on this website tells you the number of calories you need to maintain your weight. Just go to the website and search for "calorie calculator."

My Net Diary (www.mynetdiary.com)—This website counts calories, keeps a food log, and tells you exactly how much you need to eat to lose 1 to 2 pounds a week. It also tells you how long it will take to meet your goal with a calorie change.

The Daily Plate (www.thedailyplate.com)—Part of Livestrong.com, this website calculates calorie level based on activities. Here, you specify how much weight you want to lose.

WebMD (www.webmd.com)—A simple calculator that gives you the number of calories you need to eat every day to maintain your weight. Just go to the website and search for "metabolism calculator."

High-Fiber Foods

There are lots of delicious ways to get more fiber in your diet. The best sources are grains, vegetables, and fruits. In the following table is a list of fiber all-stars that you should try to include in your diet—at least one or two of them each day.

We offer this advice with one caveat—start slowly. If you've been eating a very refined, processed diet, you might experience diarrhea, gas, and bloating if you make a sudden and radical shift in your fiber intake. If this eating plan is a big change for you with respect to fiber, you might want to replace beans and other legumes (the rock stars of high-fiber foods) with 3 ounces of lean poultry or fish during the first week, gradually building up to the optimal levels of fiber intake of this eating plan. Also be sure and drink plenty of water to keep things moving.

When it comes to vegetables, if you remove the seeds, peels, and/or hulls from food, you lose a lot of fiber. As much as possible, stick with the whole food—don't peel carrots, tomatoes, cucumbers, and other veggies.

Fruits add lots of great fat-busting fiber to your diet, so you shouldn't avoid them. When choosing fruits to eat, go for those with the highest fiber counts, such as the ones in this table.

Good Sources of Dietary Fiber

Food	Serving Size	Grams of Fiber
Apple, fresh with skin	1 large	4.4
Artichoke	1 choke	7
Avocado, cubed	1 cup	10
Baked beans, canned/homemade	1 cup	12
Black beans, cooked	1 cup	15
Blackberries	1 cup	8
Blueberries	1 cup	4
Broccoli, steamed	1 cup	5.1
Brown rice, cooked	1 cup	3.5
Brussels sprouts	1 cup	4.1
Lentils, cooked	1 cup	15.6
Lima beans	1 cup	13.2
Oatmeal, cooked	1 cup	4.0
Pear, with skin	1 medium	5.5
Pearled barley, cooked	1 cup	6.0
Peas, cooked	1 cup	8.8
Quinoa, cooked	1 cup	5.2
Strawberries	1¼ cups	3.8
Sweet corn	1 cup	4.2
Winter squash	1 cup	5.7

Index

Numbers

A

B

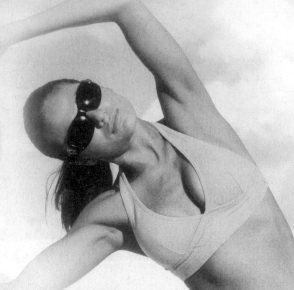
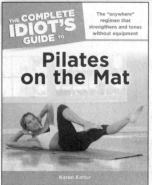
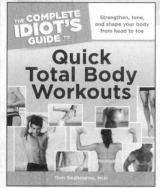
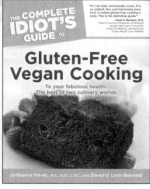
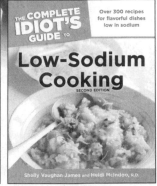
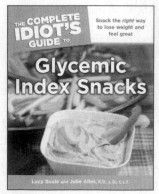
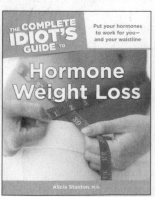
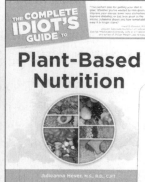
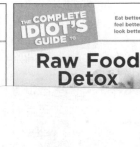

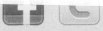